Tails from the ICU

The joy, humor, and heartache of caring for animals in crisis.

By

Andrew Linklater

Dedication

My deepest gratitude goes to all who have supported me—my family, near, far and no longer with us, and the pets who have filled my life with love.

To my colleagues in the veterinary profession, thank you for your guidance, collaboration, and encouragement throughout this journey.

Above all, this is for the animals and their devoted owners who have entrusted me with their care. Each encounter, joyful or challenging, has reminded me why I chose this path. It has been an honor to serve, to heal, and to share in so many stories of love, loss, and resilience.

Table of Content

Section 1

From Student to Specialist: Veterinary Medical Training

Chapter 1

Introduction

Well, I suppose I should start by sharing a bit about who I am and how I got here. The path into the veterinary field is different for everyone—whether you're a veterinary educator, technician, assistant, receptionist, specialist, or just a regular ol' veterinarian. For many of us, like myself, veterinary medicine is a calling—something you recognize early in life and feel compelled to pursue. For others, the journey may not be so clear-cut. It might be a second career or something discovered along the way during their education. As for me, I first recognized my calling to become a veterinarian in the second grade—well, sort of.

My second-grade teacher, Mrs. Senior, had assigned each of us a project to present to the class. The topic I chose was orcas (or "killer whales," as they were commonly known at the time). I studied them and quickly fell in love. Back then, orcas were portrayed as one of the beauties of the sea—a symbol of nature and all that was good in the world. As time went on and more research was done, that image became a bit more realistic—and a bit more gruesome. Orcas are now understood to be apex predators, often hunting seals, sharks, and even other whales.

Back to my second-grade project: if I remember correctly, my poster board presentation featured pictures I had cut out of my parents' encyclopedias. I don't think they were particularly thrilled about that part. I also realize that cutting pictures from encyclopedias really dates me—but hey, we used what we had back then. Let's move on from that, shall we? From that moment on, I was hooked on animals, and my interest in marine biology was off to a strong start.

Growing up in the landlocked province of Saskatchewan, Canada, my lack of access to local killer whales quickly became obvious, and my dream of becoming a marine biologist gradually shifted toward veterinary medicine. Below, you'll see some pictures from my early childhood. There's a photo of me with a random black dog I must have liked (Figure 1)—I look absolutely ecstatic, though I'm not sure the dog felt the same way. Then, there's a picture of my best childhood friend, a yellow Labrador mix named Buffy (Figure 2). My parents and friends shared stories for years about the bond Buffy and I shared. The one I remember most vividly is how she refused to eat unless I fed her by hand—and I was more than happy to oblige.

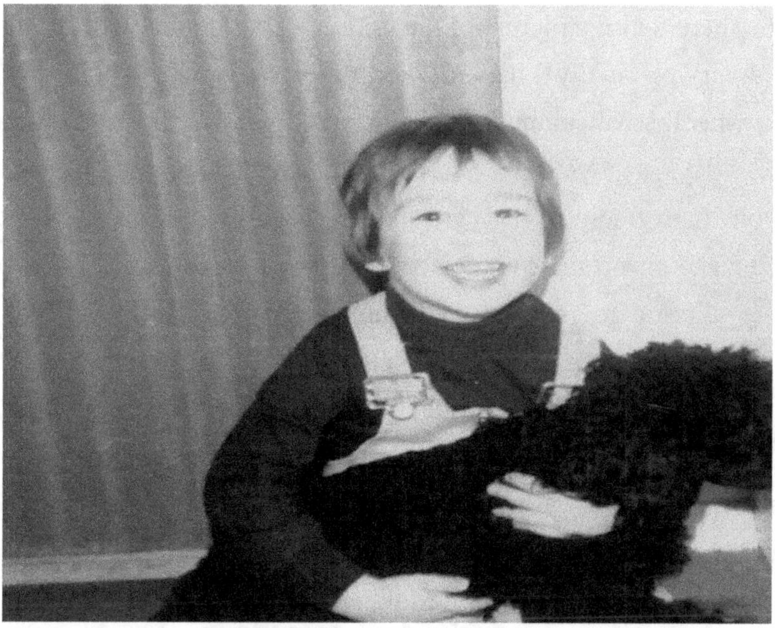

Figure 1. Loving Animals

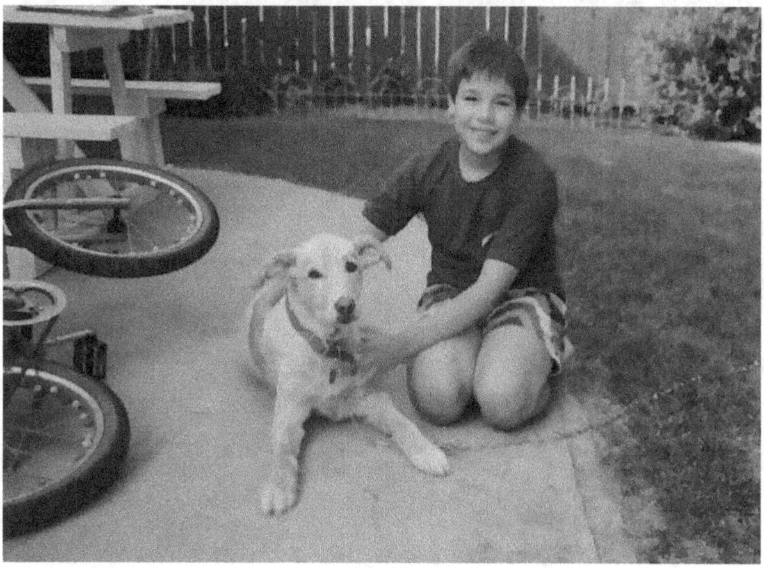

Figure 2. My First Best Friend

There's also a picture of me with my childhood rabbit, creatively (and very originally!) named Thumper. I was giving Thumper a ride in a wheelbarrow alongside one of my childhood friends (Figure 3). These days, as a veterinarian, I would never recommend letting a pet rabbit roam freely in the yard like we used to—too many stories of escapes or unfortunate encounters with predators. Ironically, I'm now quite allergic to rabbits, so I can't keep them as pets, and they certainly pose some unique challenges when I treat them in practice. But those are stories for another time.My interest in animals—and my exposure to them—continued throughout my childhood. One standout memory was getting to meet and hold a tiger cub when I was quite young. As I recall, the photo of me with the tiger cub (Figure 4) was taken at West Edmonton Mall, which I believe still holds the title of the largest mall in the world. This was back in the early '80s, and I'm pretty sure experiences like that are no longer allowed—and for good reason. Allowing the general public to interact with non-domesticated species poses serious risks, and there have been far too many tragic stories of what can go wrong when wild animals are kept by private individuals. Much of this was highlighted in the popular Netflix series *Tiger King*.

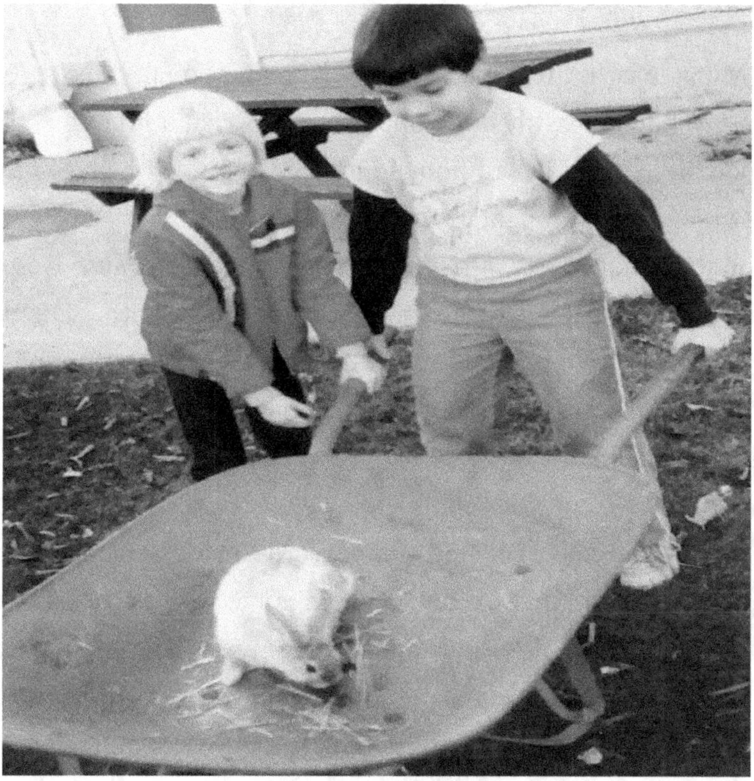

Figure 3. Thumper

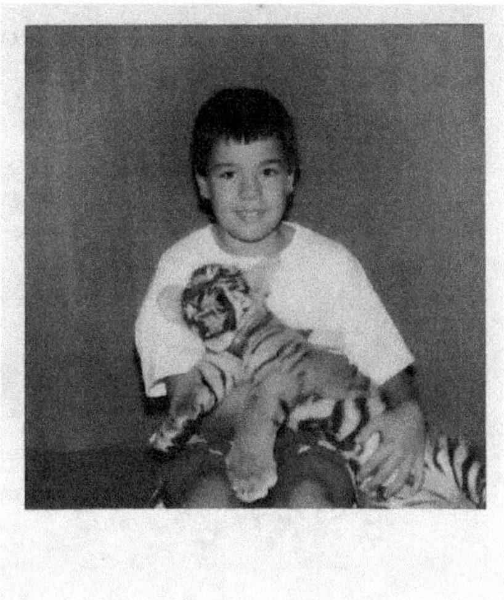

Figure 4. Tiger Baby

Much later in life, I made it a personal mission to travel to South Africa. While there, I had the opportunity to visit a lion sanctuary—an incredible place where lions injured or at risk of being killed by local villagers are brought to recover and live in safety. Of course, the reason these lions were at risk in the first place is because we pesky humans continue to encroach on their natural territories. Sanctuaries like this one rely in part on tourism to fund their efforts, and visitors like myself help provide a source of income to feed and care for these magnificent animals. In hindsight, it probably wasn't the safest thing I've ever done—but I was completely "gaga" over these lions. During that visit, I had one of my all-time favorite photos taken with them (Figures 5 and 6).Finally, pictured here is me with the second dog I ever owned (the third for our family) and my rock for many years—my emotional support companion, a golden retriever named Jasper (Figure 7). And yes, that is some fantastic brown shag carpet in the background! My family got Jasper when I was in the early years of high school, and she stayed by my side through my undergraduate studies and most of veterinary school. I used to walk her every day during my paper route—a job I held for a little over seven years.

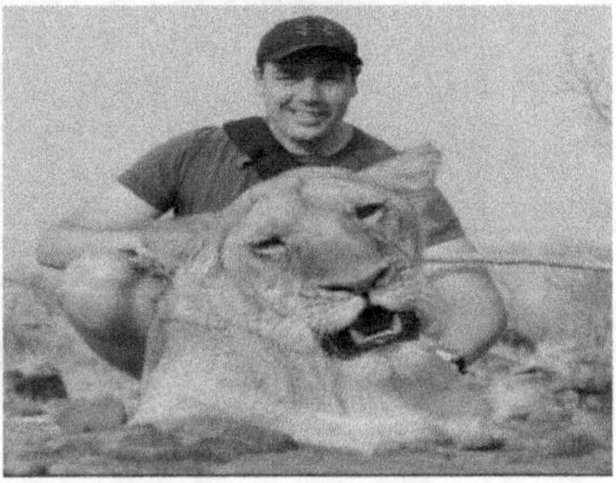

Figure 5. Lion King

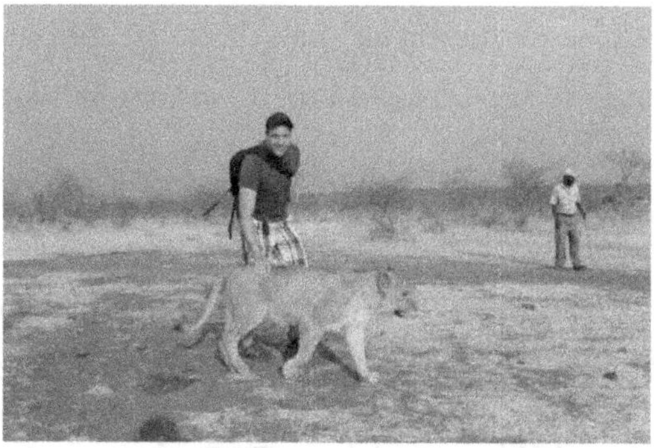

Figure 6. Lion Queen

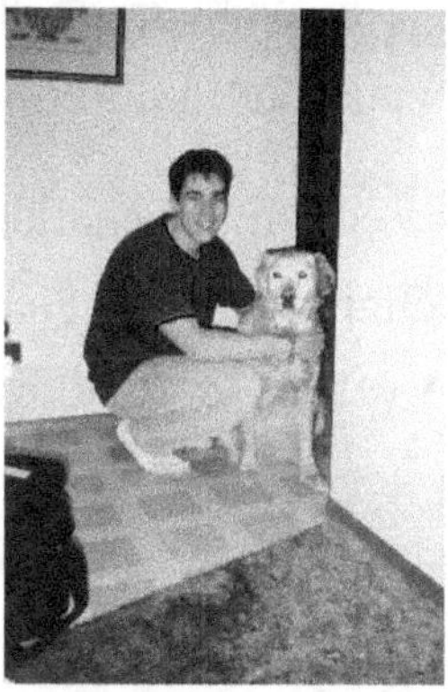

Figure 7. My Rock Jasper

Jasper was the first pet I had to say goodbye to as an adult—the first I had to euthanize—and her loss was one of the most significant of my life at that time. That kind of deep bond is something many of us share. I'm sure many of you have had that one special animal—the one who listened without judgment, who you could hug or snuggle, cry with, and share countless joyful moments. That bond can be powerful, healing, and life-changing.

Today, we understand so much more about the human-animal bond—not just emotionally, but scientifically. Research continues to show how these connections can help people with neurological disorders, anxiety, seizures, and many other challenges.

One of the biggest challenges any aspiring veterinarian faces early in their journey is getting accepted into veterinary school. Most veterinarians take great pride in the fact that admission into veterinary medical programs is notoriously competitive—often more so than other professional schools, including traditional medical (i.e., human medical) schools. Statistically speaking, your average veterinarian may even outperform your average physician in terms of academic achievement simply because getting into vet school is *that* difficult.

And it only seems to get more challenging each year. I hear this all the time from our technical staff—at least once a year, one of them is preparing to apply to veterinary school and feeling the pressure of just how tough it is to get in.Most veterinarians might even brag—just a little—about the fact that *real* doctors treat more than one species! During veterinary school, it's almost a rite of passage to see this phrase printed on coffee mugs, T-shirts, or other paraphernalia sold to raise money for various events—whether it's a class trip, a school project, or the graduation ceremony itself.

Getting into veterinary school is no small feat, and it often requires deciding on your career path very early in life. From elementary school through high school and into college, you have to work hard at every level. Your grades need to be top-tier, and you also need significant hands-on experience with animals before most veterinary schools will even consider your application. In those early years—elementary, middle, and high school—you typically need to be among the top of your class. Then comes your undergraduate education, usually a four-year degree in biology, animal science, agriculture, or a related field. During that time, your main focus is completing the prerequisite courses required for vet school applications. And once you're accepted, you're in for another four intense, grueling years of veterinary school.

Four years of challenging coursework, constant exams, and nonstop studying—that's veterinary school. During that time, you're learning how to examine, diagnose, and treat hundreds of medical conditions across thousands of different species. While most veterinarians end up focusing on farm animals (like horses, cows, pigs, sheep, and chickens) or companion animals (such as dogs, cats, and pocket pets), we're still expected to have a working knowledge of a vast array of species that we may encounter throughout our careers.

In recent decades, most veterinary schools have adopted a "tracking" system, allowing students to tailor part of their education to their area of interest. Typically, this means focusing on either small/companion animals (like dogs and cats) or large/farm animals (like horses and livestock). Some students take it further, specializing in unique areas such as avian medicine, exotic species (reptiles and amphibians), aquatic animals, or even roles within the food production industry (focusing on pigs or poultry, for example).

Regardless of the chosen path, it's a daunting challenge to absorb and master all the required knowledge in just four years. But once completed, graduates earn the title Doctor of Veterinary Medicine, or DVM—a credential awarded by most veterinary schools. There are a few regional variations: for example, in Pennsylvania, graduates of the University of Pennsylvania receive a VMD, while in many European countries, the equivalent degree is titled Master of Veterinary Science (MVS) or something similar.By the time you complete veterinary school, the average veterinarian has undergone at least 20 years of education—though that doesn't include the most important year of all: kindergarten! But the journey isn't over yet. Before you can begin practicing medicine, you must pass a national licensing exam. The North American Veterinary Licensing Examination, or NAVLE, is administered to all veterinary students by schools accredited by the American Veterinary Medical Association (AVMA).

The NAVLE is a lengthy and comprehensive exam covering everything you've learned about veterinary medicine across all species. Passing this exam is required before you can apply for a state or provincial veterinary medical license to practice. Additionally, many jurisdictions require candidates to pass a state or provincial exam, which typically focuses on local laws and region-specific infectious diseases. Only after completing these steps are you officially licensed to practice veterinary medicine in that area.

However, some veterinarians choose to further their education by specializing in a particular field.

After veterinary school, about ten percent of graduates choose to pursue an internship. This is an additional year of training, usually focused on your area of interest—small or large animals—where you gain more hands-on experience under the mentorship of various specialists before practicing independently. The most common internship is a rotating one, where you cycle through different specialty services such as internal medicine, surgery, oncology, emergency care, and more. You typically spend a few weeks on each service, giving you a broad overview of the common cases veterinarians encounter.

Of those who complete an internship, roughly ten percent go on to pursue a specialty and become "board-certified specialists."

Many people assume that veterinary specialists choose to focus on a particular species—like dogs—or even a specific breed, such as Golden Retrievers. That's simply not the case. A veterinary specialist is someone who has completed advanced and intensive training in a specific medical field, such as Internal Medicine, Surgery, Oncology, or Cardiology.

Becoming a board-certified specialist requires an additional 3 to 5 years of dedicated study and work beyond veterinary school. This includes completing a residency program that typically lasts three or more years, publishing a scientific paper in a peer-reviewed journal, and successfully passing a rigorous, multi-day certification examination. These exams are challenging, with an average annual pass rate of about 50%.

Most specialty boards now require ongoing education, and many specialists must demonstrate continued learning and professional contributions through a re-credentialing process every 10 years. My specialty is emergency and critical care, and I have completed each of these steps, earning the title of Diplomate of the American College of Veterinary Emergency and Critical Care—DACVECC for short.

I've always joked with my nieces and nephews that I was still in "Grade 24" by the time I finished school. It sounds a bit daunting to those just graduating high school—that they might only be halfway through their education!

As of 2024, according to the American Veterinary Medical Association, there are about 127,000 veterinarians practicing in the U.S. across various fields. The majority work in clinical practice directly treating animals. Others are employed in research, government positions, the military, and academia. About ten percent of veterinarians are specialists, roughly 12,000 individuals.

Would you believe the gender ratio is about two females for every male? Current graduating classes often consist of 75% or more females. As of 2020, there were approximately 800 specialists in my field of emergency and critical care. That may seem like a small number, but when I first became a specialist, there were only about 300 in the entire field. At one point after my residency, I considered moving back to Canada, where I would have been one of only three people with those credentials in the whole country. However, I decided to stay in Wisconsin after completing my residency—and I've had quite a life here!

I feel incredibly lucky to be part of the veterinary field for so many reasons. I've had the support of family, friends, and mentors who helped me through school. I get to help animals and their families every day, and I've witnessed countless humorous and amazing moments throughout my career—many of which I'll share in this book. So, let's embark on this adventure together, shall we?

Chapter 2

Things we do to get into veterinary school – meeting some inmates

As I mentioned earlier, it's hard to get into veterinary school. There are several key requirements which need to be to met. First and foremost: good grades and completion of prerequisite courses. I understand it's not a perfect system—grades don't always reflect true intelligence—but veterinary schools need a starting point to narrow down the pool of applicants, and this is usually where it begins.

Most (though not all) veterinary schools also require an in-person interview. This is a valuable step in the process because it allows applicants to demonstrate interpersonal skills and the ability to communicate clearly with others. It has always surprised me that not every veterinary school includes an interview in its admissions process—especially since interacting with people is a fundamental part of the job. As veterinarians, we have interviews with clients every day, and we're often tasked with explaining complex medical information in a way that makes sense.

Finally, one of the most important things you need to be considered for admission is a broad range of experience within the veterinary field. This helps ensure you truly understand what the profession involves.

Experience in the veterinary field is essential. Some candidates come in with a lot of it—perhaps a parent was a veterinarian, or they grew up on a farm. Some have attended veterinary technical school, while others work or volunteer in veterinary practices. Still others gain experience through volunteering at animal shelters, humane societies, or even meat packing plants. These experiences are crucial for developing a realistic understanding of what veterinary medicine truly involves—not just the romanticized version many people imagine. Far too often, people think we just play with puppies and kittens all day. In reality, it's a tough, emotional profession where critical decisions must be made every single day.

I took the volunteer route, gaining experience at a number of places: a veterinary clinic (of course), the veterinary school (thanks to a close family friend who was studying there), a wild animal rescue group, and even the local zoo. But as a city kid, I also needed some large animal experience, so I spent some volunteer hours at a nearby horse ranch.

It's especially important to get exposure to large animals if you didn't grow up on a farm. I was definitely a city kid, and stepping into various large animal situations pushed me out of my comfort zone. But that's often viewed as a positive by veterinary schools—it shows adaptability and a willingness to take on challenges.

Because of the history and storied tradition of veterinary medicine (with James Herriot being a favorite author among many future vets), I imagined myself becoming a mixed-animal practitioner—someone who works with both large and small animals—probably based in rural Saskatchewan. Despite the long, bitter winters of central Canada, that was the vision I had for a while. Well, clearly that plan didn't quite work out, but I'm truly happy doing what I do now at a specialty center. And maybe it's for the best that I mostly treat patients who weigh less than I do (with some rare exceptions). At least there's a lower—though not zero—risk of serious injury or long-term orthopedic issues when working with small animals!

My volunteering journey began at a local ranch and horse boarding facility just outside the booming Canadian metropolis of Saskatoon, Saskatchewan. Saskatoon, the largest city in the province, currently has a population of about 250,000 people. While it offers many features of a "big city," it's also surrounded by rural communities and farmland, making it an ideal place to gain experience with large animals.

The ranch where I volunteered housed both purebred riding horses and rescue animals. They welcomed volunteers, and my time there gave me invaluable hands-on exposure to horses and their behavior. I worked alongside several ranch hands doing everything from turning the horses out to their outdoor paddocks, exercising them with light riding, mucking (cleaning) stalls, feeding, organizing tack, and much more.

I particularly remember one very large horse named Big Ben. He was named after the famous horse ridden by Canadian Olympic show jumper Ian Millar—often affectionately referred to as "Captain Canada." Ian Millar is one of the most enduring Olympic athletes in history, holding the record for the most Olympic appearances by any athlete, having competed in 10 Summer Games, with his last being the 2012 London Olympics. The original Big Ben was an impressive 17.3 hands tall—over five and a half feet at the shoulder—and the Big Ben I worked with at the ranch was no different. Please don't ask me why horses are measured in "hands" rather than feet, meters, or any other normal unit of measurement… that's a mystery for another day.

The Big Ben I cared for was a gentle giant—anyone could handle him easily—but he had one very annoying habit. After I'd spent a long time cleaning out his stall, putting in fresh food and water, and letting him out for some exercise, I'd bring him back in at the end of the day… and the first thing he'd do was immediately pee. Like, a lot. And let me tell you—horse urine smells *bad*. I don't know if you've ever had the pleasure of smelling horse pee, but using the words of Ron Burgundy from the movie *Anchorman*, "It really stings the nostrils."

If you've ever smelled cat urine, you already know it's pungent and seems to seep into everything. Now imagine that—except in gallons (or liters, if you're using SI units). That was Big Ben's signature move. Every time.

Anyway, back to the ranch. Because some of the horses were rescues, the ranch had to be frugal, watching operating costs closely. To help with that, they utilized a number of cost-saving measures—including labor. Some of the work wasn't exactly done by volunteers in the traditional sense. The ranch participated in a work-release program with the local penitentiary, which meant prisoners were bussed in for a few hours each afternoon to muck the stalls. It wasn't glamorous work, but it was necessary, and I suppose for the prisoners, it was a break from being behind bars—maybe even something they looked forward to.

I had been volunteering at the ranch for several weeks when I began regularly seeing the work-release crew. Over time, I met and chatted with a few of them—though there were never any formal introductions, of course. One guy stood out in particular: a towering Native American man named Ernest. He must have weighed over 300 pounds and stood at least 6'6". You couldn't miss him.

Ernest—though most people just called him Ernie—seemed to be the leader of the group of guys that came to the ranch. Or maybe the others were just scared of him. I couldn't really tell. I was a scrawny 16-year-old kid at the time, pretty naïve to the ways of the world, so all of that was a bit over my head. Since there weren't many people around the ranch to talk to, I ended up spending a bit of time with the work-release guys, just shootin' the breeze during breaks. Horse work is no joke—it's tough labor, especially in the summer—so you've got to pause now and then, cool off, and grab some water.

One day after mucking out a particularly nasty stall, I came home and shared a few stories from the ranch with my family. I was chatting with my mom and brother, casually telling them about the horses and the routine. I eventually let slip a detail I hadn't shared before: the work-release program. I figured if I'd told them that part upfront, they might've freaked out—so I held off. But now that I'd been there a while and it seemed no big deal, I told them about some of the guys, including this one big guy named Ernest that I'd been talking to here and there.

What I hadn't considered at the time was that my mom worked as an emergency room nurse in the "not-so-nice" part of town, and my brother was a police officer in the city. They both had a pretty strong sense of "who was who" in the local scene.

They both screamed at the same time, "**Ernie??? You're working with Ernie??**" Not exactly a common name, so I figured it couldn't be a coincidence. They asked me to describe him, and as I rattled off the details—his towering height, Native heritage, and massive frame—their faces confirmed it. Yep. Same Ernie.

Turns out, Ernie had quite the reputation around the city. My mom knew him because he was notorious for faking illness to get admitted to the hospital during the frigid winter months. A warm bed, a hot meal, and some human interaction? Not a bad deal if you're trying to survive a brutal Saskatchewan winter. Meanwhile, my brother—who was a police officer—had actually arrested Ernie several times over the years, mostly for minor (thankfully, non-violent) offenses like breaking and entering.

The next week at the ranch, I struck up a conversation with some of the other guys in the work-release program. I learned that committing minor crimes like B&E wasn't all that uncommon among people facing housing insecurity. If you pulled off the "right" crime at the "right" time, you could spend the winter indoors—in jail. As harsh as that sounds, it was still better than freezing to death on the streets of central Canada in January.

Now, I'm fairly confident Ernie had done more in his time than what he let on. But I wasn't there to judge, and I definitely wasn't going to pry. He was always decent to me—cordial, helpful, even kind—and that was enough.

Spending time with the inmates at the ranch turned out to be meaningful to me in more ways than I expected. Sure, I got my volunteer hours and checked the box for large animal experience—critical components for my veterinary school application, and probably the most important things in my mind at the time. But looking back now, that experience has taken on a deeper significance.

Over the years, I've become a much more compassionate, empathetic, and understanding person, especially toward those who are less fortunate. I've been incredibly lucky in my life—always having a roof over my head, food on the table, and everything I've truly needed. But I've come to understand that this isn't the reality for everyone. People can end up in difficult, even desperate, situations that push them to make choices you might never expect if you haven't walked in their shoes.

What I learned at the ranch—beyond horses and hard labor—was a lesson in humanity. And I carry that with me still.

Chapter 3

Learnin' 'bout the burnin'

I'm not going to apologize for some of the gruesome things I'm about to share in this book—but consider this your fair warning: there are plenty of stories that get a little gross, and occasionally, downright graphic. These are the kinds of things that happen in veterinary clinics all the time—it's just part of the job. Many aspects of biology are messy, so try not to be too surprised. The good news? This book doesn't come with "smell-o-vision," so you won't be subjected to some of the truly awful odors we deal with. But make no mistake—there are certain smells that every veterinary professional knows all too well.

Thankfully, I don't have the strongest sense of smell, which works in my favor. But odors are a constant part of life in a veterinary clinic. Sure, you've got the usual suspects like stool (feces, poo, dookie—whatever term you prefer), but it can get much worse. Think: anal glands, abscesses, or the unmistakable scent of rotting or burning flesh and bone. Okay, that might sound a little extreme—but in small doses, this is regular fare in our line of work. And I'll explain why very soon.

When you enter any medical profession—especially nowadays—you slowly come to realize that you've probably lived a relatively sheltered life. Most likely, your parents did their best to minimize your exposure to things that are scary, perverse, or just plain gross.

It's tough to learn about these things as you start encountering the real world, but the unpleasant parts of life are facts we all have to process as we move into adulthood.

The good news is, I'm not going to describe anything too "out there" here—just some of the realities of life.

Many things we learn as kids—like everyone poops. It's a basic necessity we all deal with. Mostly it's normal, sometimes it's gross, but everyone does it. Everyone vomits too—and that's really gross. Most of us feel terrible when it happens. My wife actually has a strong aversion to vomiting; even hearing the sounds or seeing it on TV makes her cringe. I don't think anyone really likes it. But at the veterinary hospital, vomiting is a regular occurrence. Sometimes, it's not all that bad—like when we induce vomiting in a dog that's eaten a large amount of chocolate. Oddly enough, that actually smells pretty good! Figure 8 shows a dog vomiting after chocolate ingestion. This was a relatively small amount, and there were no wrappers involved.

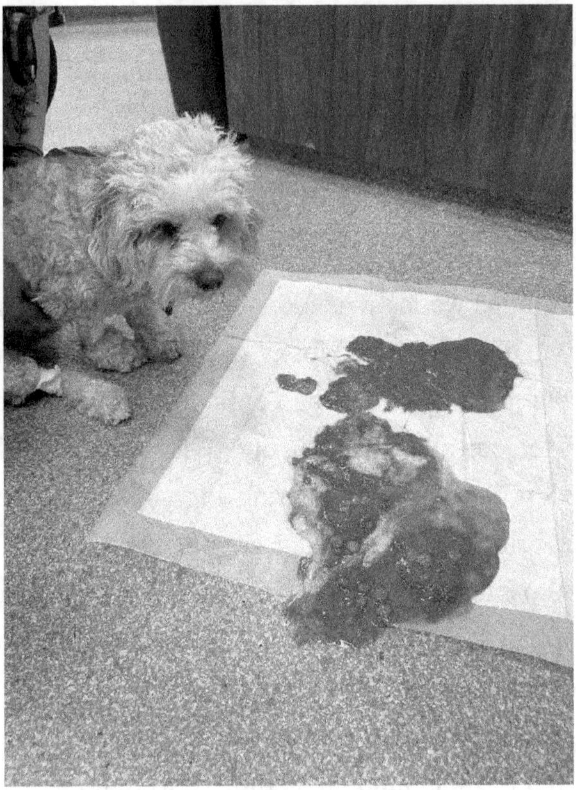

Figure 8. Choclate Vomit

There are no pictures for the next couple of stories—I figured the descriptions of the smells will be nasty enough!I first started volunteering at a neighborhood veterinary clinic to gain more veterinary exposure before applying to vet school. One of the local clinics belonged to a family friend, known to my parents through my older brother's hockey coaches—a truly Canadian connection. "Dr. G" was his name, and he became my first official veterinary mentor. He was a small animal primary care practitioner at a clinic within walking distance of my childhood home.

One day, I called Dr. G at his clinic and asked if I could volunteer on Saturday mornings. Luckily for me, he was more than happy to oblige, encouraging a young aspiring veterinarian like myself to enter the profession. Saturday mornings at most veterinary clinics aren't terribly busy, usually just a half-day. Most of the appointments are what I like to call "convenience appointments"—mostly vaccinations or routine health checks. Saturday morning hours are often the only option for people who work Monday to Friday and need to get their pets seen.

So, for a couple of years, most of my Saturday mornings were spent for a few hours at the clinic. One Saturday morning, however, was a bit more unusual. When I arrived, several appointments had been cancelled, leaving some open time. The first client asked if the doctor could perform a dental procedure, and Dr. G agreed. The animal was sedated and placed under general anesthesia, while being carefully monitored. Dental x-rays revealed a fractured molar that needed to be extracted.

So, out came the drill. Anyone who's been near a dental drill knows that high-pitched "weeeeeeeeeeeeeeeeeeee" sound that makes most people cringe—I'm definitely one of them. I've always hated the dentist. The noise instantly triggers that familiar internal panic, and I start sweating a little. Maybe I'm not alone—there must be a lot of you out there who feel the same kind of anxiety! That sound might have been the first thing to make me uneasy that morning. Or maybe it was how limp the dog went after being put under anesthesia. I'm not sure, but I leaned in closer, too curious to look away.The doctor had me put on gloves and a mask so he could show me a few things. And then, things got a little worse for me. The latex gloves trapped heat on my hands, making them sweat even more. Inside the surgical mask, I was breathing on my own face—something we've all become painfully familiar with since the pandemic—and that only added to my discomfort. Everything was getting warmer, sweatier, and a whole lot more uncomfortable.I moved in closer to get a better idea of what was happening. The doctor explained that canine teeth are quite different from human teeth. Some of the larger ones need to be cut into pieces before removal because they have multiple, very large roots. Besides the drilling, a lot of constant, significant force must be applied to the periodontal ligament to break it down, which allows the tooth to come out.

The next thing that made me uneasy was the visual. He placed a periosteal elevator into the dog's mouth—a large, cold, steel instrument—and pushed it so hard against the dog's gums that it looked like he was about to break the dog's jaw. Most surgical instruments look a little like medieval torture devices (go ahead, Google "periosteal elevator" if you want to see what I mean).

Of course, he wasn't going to break the dog's jaw, but if you had never seen it before, it would definitely make you uneasy. For me, it made me a little queasy… and probably a bit sweatier too. It felt like someone had cranked up the thermostat, and the room got noticeably hotter.

Then came the drill again, with that high-pitched "weeeeeeeeeeeeeeeeeeeeeeeeee" sound.

A minute or two later, what really "tipped me over the edge" — and hit me like a ton of bricks — was the smell. This particular odor is one you never forget once you've experienced it: burning bone (or, in this case, burning tooth). It's a tough smell to describe—kind of like burning hair, but somehow worse. It's not something most people encounter very often.

Your best chance of smelling burning bone might be at the dentist, but most dentists use an air suction device to whisk the smell away quickly. Even in the worst case, human dental patients only catch subtle hints of it. That's not how it works in a veterinary clinic.

Suddenly, I was painfully aware of how hot I felt—from the smell, the heat, the pressure on the jaw—and the room started to spin. I could feel the blood draining from my face. The doctor looked up, clearly noticing my pale complexion, and said, "Go sit down and put your head between your knees." I did just that.

I sat down with my head between my knees, peeling off my mask and gloves. Gradually, the room stopped spinning, and I started to feel a little better. The technician kindly brought me some water, which helped even more. Luckily, I didn't pass out — but I was close. That experience, and that unforgettable smell, have stayed with me ever since.

Maybe that moment was part of why I ended up in emergency medicine. Emergency vets rarely deal with dental procedures, and when we do, it's usually just a temporary fix. I basically don't handle dental emergencies unless they're painful, broken, or infected — in which case the patient gets pain medications, antibiotics and a referral back to their primary care veterinarian. I'm happy to leave that awful burning bone smell to someone else.

To this day, I still don't like going to the dentist. My hands start sweating, and it's a good thing I'm already lying down when I'm there!

Chapter 4

Why we get into veterinary medicine

There's no single reason why someone becomes a veterinarian. Veterinary medicine is highly romanticized—ask around, and even if you don't personally know a veterinarian, I can almost guarantee you know someone who wanted to be one, still wants to be one, or has a child who dreams of becoming one. There's something undeniably idyllic about veterinarians. Maybe it's the gentle, caring hand. Maybe it's the idea of helping animals—something many of us feel instinctively drawn to. Maybe it's the appeal of being a doctor. More likely, it's a combination of all those things.

But one thing I can tell you for certain—and nearly every veterinarian would agree: we do *not* get into this profession for the money. In fact, quite the opposite.

Most veterinarians graduate with significant, sometimes crippling, student loan debt. At the time of this writing, tuition alone at most veterinary schools runs into the tens of thousands of dollars per year. That doesn't even include the cost of books, housing, food, supplies, and other living expenses. The average debt upon graduation is well into six figures, and those loans often take decades to repay.

We face the same level of debt as physicians going through medical school, yet we typically earn *less than half* the salary of a primary care MD. (Don't take my word for it—just Google it. This information is widely available now.)

That's also why we have to charge for our services. Veterinary clinics have staff, equipment, facilities, and yes, even our own paychecks to cover. And once we get paid, much of that income goes toward the same expenses everyone else has—mortgage or rent, groceries, taxes, gas, insurance—but a huge chunk also goes straight to repaying student loans. For many veterinarians, loan payments stretch over the course of an entire career.This is something I feel strongly about—educating people on the realities of veterinary finances. Ask anyone about their most recent trip to the vet, and if it's not the first thing they mention, it's usually the second: the cost.

"I took my dog to the vet last week because he was vomiting, and the bill was over $500!"

We hear it all the time.

The truth is, many of our staff members make just above minimum wage, despite their incredible skill sets. And let me be clear: veterinarians could not do our jobs without them. Skilled veterinary technicians and support staff are absolutely essential to everything we do. They take on critical responsibilities—administering medications, monitoring anesthesia, assisting in surgery, communicating with clients—and yet their compensation often doesn't reflect the value they bring.

Even so, veterinary medicine consistently operates at a fraction of the cost of human healthcare. For example, a major abdominal surgery at a veterinary hospital—such as the removal of a tumor—

might cost anywhere from $5,000 to $7,000. That exact same procedure in a human hospital could cost ten to twenty times more.For me, going to veterinary school wasn't just a goal—it was something I had always wanted to do. Or more accurately, something I had always wanted to be. You couldn't have convinced me otherwise. For many in this profession, being a veterinarian isn't just an occupation—it's an identity. It defines who we are as people. Whether we become veterinarians or we're simply born to be veterinarians is up for debate, but for some of us, the calling is undeniable.

I've already mentioned how my childhood dream of becoming a marine biologist began with a second-grade project on orcas. Over time, that dream gradually evolved into a passion for caring for all animals—and from that point on, I never looked back. I spent the next 12 years gaining experience, developing my skills, and working hard in school to pursue the dream I knew I was meant to follow.Now, I oversee a critical care service at a multi-specialty emergency and referral center. For the past 15 years or so, I've also been reviewing letters from applicants to our internship program.

Unlike many fields in human medicine, internships are not required for veterinarians, and in fact, most choose not to pursue one.

Some graduates opt out simply because they're "done" being students—though truthfully, in this profession, we're always students to some degree. Others may want to start a family, which has often been delayed for many years while working to get into and through veterinary school. Unfortunately, a far more common reason these days is the weight of student debt. With such high financial burdens, many graduates feel the pressure to begin earning a living right away rather than taking on an additional year of relatively low-paid internship training.

Regardless of the path that a veterinarian takes in their career, there is almost always two unmistakable and remarkably common themes of veterinarians: *the human-animal bond and a spirit of service*:"My mom/dad was a veterinarian, and I was always excited by the late evening call ins…I'd get to go to work with my parent and see what they did…."

"I always had a love for animals growing up…."

"I had animals growing up…"

"My first job was a kennel assistant at the humane society or a veterinary clinic and I saw how animals could be helped…"

"I've always wanted to help families with difficult decisions…"

"I volunteered at the local animal shelter where I first developed a close relationship with animals…"

For each veterinarian, the desire may be different…but we are all caring people and want to help varying aspect of our community; companion animals obviously, however we also help with world health: One Health, herds and community health, food and fiber sources and more. We are all so interconnected and so often veterinarians are a vital part to our current society.

So, be kind to your veterinarian and their staff! There is always good intent and we always and continually strive to help our clients patients as best as we can at a reasonable cost.

Chapter 5

Field trips and factory tours

Who doesn't love a school field trip, right? Some of the best memories from childhood involve those special days—visiting the local nature preserve, sports complex, science center, or, if you were really lucky, even the movie theatre or the local pool. Parents had to sign permission slips, and it felt like an exciting "day off" from the usual routine of schoolwork.

Those were truly special days. If it was a *really* good day, you even got to pack a lunch—or maybe there was a pizza party waiting for you at your destination. As school kids, we always had fun on those trips. Maybe we learned something... maybe not. But it was always a good time!What great memories we made on those days—breaking away from the humdrum of school (or, later in life, work) for a literal field day.Well, things aren't quite so happy-go-lucky when it comes to veterinary school field trips—but yes, we have them. Unfortunately, these trips aren't about fun; they're purely educational. And by educational, I mean the kind that burns images into your brain you'll never be able to unsee. And forget about packing a sack lunch—you'd be lucky not to *lose* your lunch.

I suppose that's part of what "adulting" is all about: realizing that a field trip as a kid is a wildly different experience than one as an adult.

If I may digress for a moment—think about going to Disney. As a kid, it's pure magic: fun, games, treats, rides, and adventure! But as an adult? It's a frustrating drive, a battle for parking, and a constant hemorrhaging of money in a crowded, noisy park that smells vaguely like hot asphalt, churros and sweat. You spend your day standing in long lines, only to leave with a headache, an empty bank account, and a mild case of existential dread while fighting traffic all the way home.

Field trips in veterinary school? Definitely the adult version of that.

Where do we go on these so-called "educational outings"? Well, some aren't so bad—like visits to farms, where we learn how animals are vaccinated and dewormed. Or that first time you visit a milking parlor and realize how well dairy cows can be cared for. Or a trip to a research facility, where scientists are developing new medications and vaccines. Those trips are educational *and* actually kind of fun.Then there are the field trips that are *not* so much fun… and probably part of the reason there are so many vegetarian (or vegan) veterinarians. What follows is a brief account of the two most horrific field trips I took during veterinary school.

First up: the rendering plant.

If you don't know what rendering is… please, don't Google it. Trust me—you won't like what you find. But I'll do my best to describe it here.

Rendering is actually a necessary part of modern society, and I'll explain why.

During the process of slaughtering animals for food, there are certain parts that no one wants to eat and that aren't suitable for pet food or other manufacturing uses. In addition, some animals—like cows—may die from natural causes, such as an infection, and their meat becomes unsafe for human or animal consumption. These animals are not allowed to enter the food chain.

Another example? Roadkill. Imagine a deer hit by a car and left to sit, rotting in the hot summer sun for a week or two (or longer) before being picked up by provincial or county workers. Sometimes, if the animal isn't too decomposed, parts of it might be salvaged and used to feed animals at a local zoo. But often, that's not a viable option.

Something has to be done with these bodies—and that's where rendering comes in.

Even spoiled meat from grocery stores or restaurant waste may be sent to a rendering facility. It's not glamorous, but it's a practical—and essential—solution for dealing with animal remains that can't be used in any other way.The whole point of rendering is to extract something useful from what most of us would consider completely useless—and while it's a successful and important process, it's not one most people want to think about, let alone discuss over dinner. Still, as unpleasant as it may be, rendering is a necessary part of modern life.

We're all pretty comfortable with tossing our trash into a plastic- or metal-lined bin, setting it out on the curb, and having it whisked away each week by a garbage truck—out of sight, out of mind. But just like recycling plastics or composting food waste, rendering is a way to repurpose animal remains into something useful.

For those of you with pets—don't worry, pets are not incorporated into the rendering process.

A friend of my sister once euthanized her dog and later texted me in a panic, asking what would happen if the pet wasn't cremated. She had read somewhere that cats and dogs were being rendered. I reassured her that this wasn't the case—companion animals are almost exclusively cremated or buried. In fact, it's illegal to incorporate pets (and humans, for that matter!) into the rendering process.

The rendering process takes whole animal remains and separates fats from bone and protein. The materials are cooked to remove moisture, then separated through mechanical or chemical processes. The end products are used in a wide variety of applications. Yes, sometimes that includes animal feed and pet food—it's a rich source of fat and protein, and a way to make use of materials most people would never willingly consume.

Depending on the quality and processing standards, some of the material may even be used for human-grade products, such as lard or other tallow-based goods. The process also helps stabilize the material, making it less prone to spoilage. Rendered fats can be used to manufacture soap, rubber, plastics, candles, and raw materials for the chemical industry. When an entire carcass is rendered, leather can be salvaged from the skin.

Here's a staggering fact: in the U.S. alone, roughly 28 million tons—or about 56 billion pounds—of bio-waste are rendered each year. Without this process, we'd be facing an enormous disposal problem.Rendering is necessary—but it's also undeniably gross. Large pieces of animals—or sometimes entire carcasses—are tossed into industrial grinders and then cooked. This all takes place on a massive scale, using giant vats. And as a veterinary student, when you're "lucky enough" to tour a rendering plant and witness (and smell) the process in all its disgusting detail, the experience tends to leave you slightly traumatized, somewhat educated, and absolutely stinky.

The smell is *potent*, *pungent*, and it *lingers*. It's not something you easily forget. That said, we should consider ourselves fortunate that there are people in society willing to take on these dirty, difficult, and essential jobs.

Learning about the many layers of a veterinary career is crucial—something I certainly didn't fully understand before entering vet school. Most people think of veterinarians as simply caregivers for pets. But the field is far broader. Veterinarians also work in zoos, public health, biomedical research, and food safety across various industries. One of our most important roles is ensuring the safety of the food supply.

That's why every veterinary student is exposed, at some point in their training, to different aspects of the food chain—especially meat, milk, and egg production. Which brings me to another unforgettable moment from vet school: our field trip to the slaughterhouse.The particular slaughterhouse we visited specialized in pigs. I suppose the more appropriate term is "meat processing plant," but let's be realistic about what happens inside these facilities. If you've ever been exposed to one, you'll understand exactly what I mean. It's like the dirty, often unspoken underbelly of our food system—something most people don't see or talk about. So here, I'm going to shine a little light on it.

This can be an emotional and controversial topic. My intention isn't to stir debate, but to share the reality of what occurs behind those walls.

In our modern society—where consuming meat is still the norm—meat packing plants are an essential part of how we live and eat. And I'll be honest: visiting one made me fully understand why some people choose to become vegetarians or vegans. Most people don't hunt, dress, preserve, and package their own meat. Instead, we rely on others to do it for us, allowing us to conveniently pick up neatly wrapped cuts from the grocery store, far removed from the realities of how it got there.

As someone with a veterinary education, I feel strongly that anyone who consumes meat should at least have a basic understanding of how it reaches their plate. The process is large-scale, industrialized, and—yes—often quite shocking.

Meat processing plants are necessary as long as humans continue to raise and consume animals. That said, slaughter should always be performed humanely and under the oversight of a licensed veterinarian to ensure ethical practices.

At the pig processing plant we toured, the animals were trucked in from finishing facilities, where they had been fed and raised for optimal weight gain. They arrived by the truckload and were moved down a chute into the facility—this is where things begin to get unpleasant.

For those who haven't seen it firsthand, euthanizing a food animal is nothing like euthanizing a pet. When a companion animal is put to sleep, it's done with the utmost care, consideration, and emphasis on comfort and minimizing stress. That is not the case in food animal processing.

At the end of the chute, the animals are rendered unconscious using a method called stunning. One common approach is with a captive bolt gun—essentially a device that delivers a strong blow to the head, resulting in immediate loss of consciousness. Other methods include gassing or electrical stunning, but the goal is always the same: to induce unconsciousness before the next step.

Once the animal is unconscious, a knife is inserted into the thoracic inlet—the area where the neck meets the chest—to sever a major artery, typically the carotid. This causes the animal to bleed out within about a minute. It is undeniably difficult to watch, but the process is considered humane by most regulatory bodies because it results in a rapid death, avoids pain during the final moments, and ensures that no chemicals enter the food chain.

After the animal has died and the majority of its blood has drained, it is hoisted by its hind legs onto a conveyor system. Often, the first stop is a scalding tank, which helps sterilize the exterior of the carcass; in some facilities, a brief singeing or torching process is used first to remove body hair. Suspended high on the conveyor, the animal then proceeds through the butchering process, where it is broken down into various marketable cuts of meat.

Before any of that, however, the internal organs are removed. While many of these organs are nutrient-rich and high in vitamins, they are largely considered inedible by Western standards and are typically processed separately.

Some parts of the animal are used for dietary supplements or processed as lower-grade meats, including tripe, tongue, liver, and more. The first step in removing the internal organs is carried out by one particularly unlucky worker perched on a high chair, operating a drill with a wide bore attachment. This person is known as the "debunger," responsible for coring out the rectum of the animal—an unpleasant but necessary task that facilitates the removal of the gastrointestinal tract.

The environment inside the facility is intense: hot, humid, and saturated with the smell of death and decomposing organ matter. It's not a place most people could even imagine visiting—let alone working in. But if you're someone who eats meat, this is a reality worth acknowledging.

As the animals move down the conveyor, the internal organs are extracted—some of which are rendered, while others are sorted for different uses. Once that step is complete, the hide is typically removed, and the carcass is quickly quartered and broken down further into smaller sections. These sections are prepared for inspection, processing, and packaging. Individual portions slide along stainless steel tables, where skilled workers (or, in some cases, machines) with sharp knives process them into cuts recognizable at the grocery store.

The lower-quality, yet still edible, parts of the animal are funneled into a grinder. The grinder's smell is distinctive—almost like that of hot dogs. Bits of meat and organs are ground, blended, and cooked in massive vats. When fully processed, this mixture becomes the base for various processed meats—hot dogs, bologna, and similar products. Appetizing, right?

Keep in mind: when a label says "100% Beef" or "100% Pork," that doesn't mean it's 100% prime muscle meat—it simply means that 100% of the ingredients came from a cow or a pig. Likely not what you pictured when you read the packaging.

The sight and smell of that plant—and especially that vat—left an impression I've never been able to shake. While I didn't become a vegan after that visit, I've certainly thought about it more seriously and have reduced my meat consumption over the years as a result. Beef, chicken, and seafood all undergo similar processes in the path from farm to fork.

It's far too easy to forget where our food comes from when it's neatly packaged in Styrofoam and shrink wrap at Costco or the local grocery store.

So, be grateful—truly grateful—that someone is willing to do this work. And if nothing else, maybe you now feel just a little more informed about what happens behind the scenes.

By the end of those two unforgettable field trips, I walked away with some powerful olfactory and visual memories—ones that will last a lifetime.

Chapter 6

The intimate association between food and a veterinarian

Or, the way to a veterinarian's heart…I obviously had some trouble coming up with a title for this particular chapter. And, once again, this might be one of those chapters that's a little graphic for some readers. If you've got a queasy stomach or can't quite handle the idea of bodily fluids and food being discussed in the same breath, this might be your cue to skip ahead to the next story. But if you've made it this far—through rendering plants and slaughterhouse field trips—you'll probably do just fine here too.

The relationship between a veterinarian and food often begins quite early in their education—typically in the first year of veterinary school—with a deceptively simple class called Comparative Anatomy. Sounds innocent enough, right? But this course is no joke. We spend countless hours learning about the body: every organ, every blood vessel, every nerve pathway. We study muscles in detail, right down to their origin and insertion points on bones. It's a deeply intricate and absolutely essential part of veterinary education. After all, if we don't learn what "normal" anatomy looks like, how can we ever hope to recognize when something has gone wrong—or fix it?

And here's a little inside joke you'll hear from just about every veterinary student: we're all pretty convinced that anatomy lab is scheduled *right before lunch* on purpose. It feels like a test—one designed to toughen us up. Think about it: you're elbow-deep in a dissection, the air thick with the unmistakable scent of preservative chemicals and exposed tissue, and just as you're finishing up… it's time to eat. Coincidence? Most of us don't think so.

Maybe the timing *is* just a fluke of scheduling, but whether intentional or not, the result is the same. Somewhere in the midst of poking around inside a cadaver and identifying anatomical landmarks, your stomach will inevitably start to growl. You'll feel hunger creeping in—even in the middle of an experience that would make most people lose their appetite. It's unsettling at first. Then, oddly enough, it becomes normal. It's a strange rite of passage in veterinary school—the beginning of what I call "taming the beast."

It's not just about getting used to the sights and smells of the job. It's about learning to compartmentalize, to manage discomfort, to keep moving even when things get unpleasant. That's a skill every veterinarian needs. Because let's face it—animals can't tell us what's wrong, and sometimes we have to go digging (sometimes literally) to figure it out.Now, some of you might imagine that anatomy lab is a very sterile environment—students in pristine lab coats, carefully examining gleaming white bones, gently pointing at bony protuberances with sanitized surgical instruments. It may start out that way, but that image quickly fades.

While technology continues to advance—and perhaps one day cadavers will become obsolete—many veterinary schools still rely on a combination of preserved and freshly deceased animal cadavers for anatomy instruction. There's just no true substitute for the tactile experience of real tissue, especially early in our training.

We're taught very early in our careers that there is much to learn from those who have died. Understanding anatomy and pathology allows us to reduce suffering and prevent future deaths. This is true in our anatomy courses and also in our pathology labs, where we learn about disease processes. Later, in clinical practice, we carry that training into post-mortem exams—or necropsies—to determine why a patient has died.

And just to ease any concerns: yes, the animals used for anatomy lab are obtained through humane, regulated, and ethical means. There are strict protocols in place to ensure this. Many of these animals are preserved in formaldehyde, allowing us to study the intricacies of muscles, nerves, and structural anatomy before ever putting hands on a living patient.

Formaldehyde is great for preserving tissues like muscle and connective tissue, but it's not as effective for organs that aren't sterile—like lungs, intestines, and other gastrointestinal structures. This is where freshly deceased cadavers are invaluable. They allow us to handle and examine organs in their most realistic state, giving us a sense of what they're supposed to feel and look like in a living, breathing animal.

Before I move on, it's worth mentioning the scope of our studies. While there's ongoing debate about how best to teach veterinary anatomy, most schools still require students to learn about *many* domestic species—not just dogs and cats, but also rabbits and horses, cows, pigs, chickens, and more. Fun fact: do you know what rabbits and horses have in common? (I'll leave that little teaser hanging.)

This wide range of species is why our course is called *Comparative Anatomy.* Rather than studying each species in isolation, we focus on the differences between them—which, surprisingly, helps us better understand the things they all share. It's a fascinating and humbling experience, and one of the core building blocks of our education. You see, human physicians have the luxury of studying just *one* species: people. Veterinarians, on the other hand, have to learn the inner workings of *everything else.* And while there are certainly similarities across species, there are just as many critical differences—especially when it comes to things like diet, digestion, anatomy, and even feces.

So, to answer that earlier question: what do rabbits and horses have in common? They're both *hindgut fermenters*, which means they derive a large portion of their nutrition from fermentation in the colon. Fascinatingly, did you know that rabbits actually eat their own stool at night? It's not as strange as it sounds—it's a vital part of their normal gastrointestinal function, helping them absorb key nutrients their bodies didn't capture the first time through.

We also pick up plenty of other fun (and sometimes bizarre) anatomical facts. For instance, did you know pigs have the most complete set of teeth among the common veterinary species? A full 44 adult teeth! Or that pigs have a spiral-shaped colon that looks oddly like a giant cinnamon roll? Yep—sometimes it's impossible *not* to relate anatomy back to food.

I digress, of course—but these kinds of facts are more than trivia. They're essential knowledge, even for veterinarians who plan to work exclusively with small animals. Every once in a while, something unexpected walks—or gets carried—through your clinic doors, and you'll need to draw on these early lessons.

When we study anatomy—particularly organs and tissues that don't preserve well—nothing beats examining a *fresh* specimen. These are samples taken directly from recently deceased animals that haven't been chemically preserved. For many veterinary species, large quantities of these tissues come from slaughterhouses.

As I discussed earlier, much of the internal anatomy from slaughtered animals is either rendered (turned into products like soap or livestock feed) or deemed unsuitable for human consumption. Some parts, however, *do* make it into the food supply—such as liver, tripe, tongue, and even feet. Personally, I find those parts hard to swallow—literally—but many people around the world love them.

And then there's the final category: organs like livers, lungs, and entire gastrointestinal systems that wind up in veterinary schools. Sometimes they arrive straight from the slaughterhouse; other times, a few days later. Either way, they're an invaluable resource for students learning to recognize what's normal—and what's not—within the inner workings of the body.I'm not quite sure how to describe the smell that comes from a gastrointestinal tract that's been sitting around for a few days. Occasionally—*occasionally*—it can be pleasant if it comes from an herbivorous species like a cow or horse. It might remind you of being outdoors on a farm or standing near the large-animal enclosure at a zoo. Maybe it even conjures the smell of freshly cut grass. Unfortunately, those fleeting earthy notes disappear quickly once these organs have been sitting for a while.

We all know the smell of rotting food, right? It's worse than that. We all know what a fart smells like, right? It's worse than that too. There's a reason, I believe, that the anatomy lab was placed at the farthest end of the building from the cafeteria.

In these labs, we don gloves and often end up with our hands—or sometimes our arms—buried up to the elbows in anatomical samples. It's not glamorous, but it's essential. And you *do* learn important lessons. For instance, most people know that cows have four stomachs, but that's not quite accurate—it's actually one stomach divided into four specialized compartments: the rumen, reticulum, omasum, and abomasum.

For me, the back end of the GI tract is where things get especially interesting. Take the tightly spiraled shape of a goat's colon, or the corkscrew structure of a pig's intestines. Or the horse's rectum—giant, complex, and oddly curvaceous. These details stick with you. Unfortunately, the *smell* sticks with you too.

In modern society, most of us are far removed from the realities of death. We don't regularly encounter the smell of decomposing internal organs. But I can tell you—it's bad. It's the kind of smell that lingers, not just in your clothes or under your fingernails, but in your nose. You might wash your hands and face, take a shower, even launder your scrubs, but the odor clings to your memory—and your sinuses—for days. Let's just say it tends to linger straight through lunch hour.

So, yes, the introduction to anatomy is pretty gross. But the grossness of veterinary medicine doesn't end there. Not by a long shot.

In first-year veterinary school, we focus on what's *normal*—healthy anatomy, normal physiology. But in the later years, we graduate to classes like *Gross Pathology.* And trust me, that name is not an exaggeration. In pathology, we learn what happens when things go wrong. Diseases, trauma, infections—basically all the ways animals can become ill or die.

A key part of that training involves performing necropsies. These post-mortem exams help us determine how and why an animal died, and most importantly, they teach us how to recognize the signs of disease so that we can diagnose, treat, and prevent it in the future.

Fun fact: Do you know the difference between a *necropsy* and an *autopsy*? A *necropsy* is a post-mortem examination performed on an animal—*any* non-human species—by a human. An *autopsy*, on the other hand, is when a human examines the body of another human after death.After we complete *gross* pathology—examining tissues with the naked eye during a necropsy—we then move to the *microscopic* level of pathology. Those same organ samples get sliced into tiny pieces so they can be examined under a microscope, helping us understand how everything functions on a cellular level as well.

In my final year of veterinary school, one particular pathology rotation left something behind with me. Actually, *on* me. And honestly… *in* me, too.

Like most days on the pathology rotation, we arrived at the lab early in the morning and gathered with our senior veterinary pathologist to review the list of animals that had passed away the previous day and were available for post-mortem examination. Each case was assigned to a student pair. Who would necropsy the dog hit by a car the night before? Who would examine the deceased cow from the Smith farm? As always, the goal was to investigate the cause of death so we could better understand disease processes and—hopefully—prevent or treat them in the future.

My "lucky" day came when personnel from a nearby provincial park (remember, I'm Canadian) brought in some long-forgotten specimens that had been left at the bottom of their freezer for *about three years*. Two of them were skunks.

The skunks had already been skinned—no one seemed to know why—and no one knew why they'd been stored that long, either. But our job was to find out why they died.

Let me tell you… the smell of a three-year-frozen, now-thawed and decomposing skunk—complete with their legendary anal scent glands—was something I'll never forget. It clung to everything: clothes, skin, nose hairs, soul.

This wasn't just your typical skunk smell. This was a decaying, fermented, freezer-burned *legacy* of stench. When we started cutting into that poor, rancid creature, the odor didn't just fill the pathology lab—it spread to the small animal clinic, the large animal clinic, and beyond. Entire portions of the hospital had to be vacated until the air could clear. And there I was… standing squarely in the eye of the storm, letting the stench settle into every fiber of my being.

I'm fairly certain that our senior pathologist later regretted the decision to assign the skunks to the student team.

No amount of showering, shampoo, or laundering (even the clothes *underneath* our protective gear) made any difference. It took a full week before the smell finally stopped lingering in my nose. And I'm sure my family—whom I was living with during vet school—thought it took much longer than that.

Oh, and yes, I performed that skunk necropsy right before lunch.

Did it stop me from eating? Not at all.

Thanks to all those lovely anatomy labs in first year, my stomach was already well-conditioned. One of the lesser-known superpowers of a veterinarian is an iron-clad appetite. After all, we spend our days working with every bodily fluid imaginable—many of which, unfortunately, have a distressing resemblance in smell, texture, or appearance to various food items. But that's a story for another chapter (and definitely not one for the squeamish).

I'm going to grab a snack before writing the next story.

And just for your entertainment, below is a picture of me (Figure 9) during one of our sheep labs, mid-procedure, extruding the penis of a ram. You can practically see the joy radiating from my face. What a day!

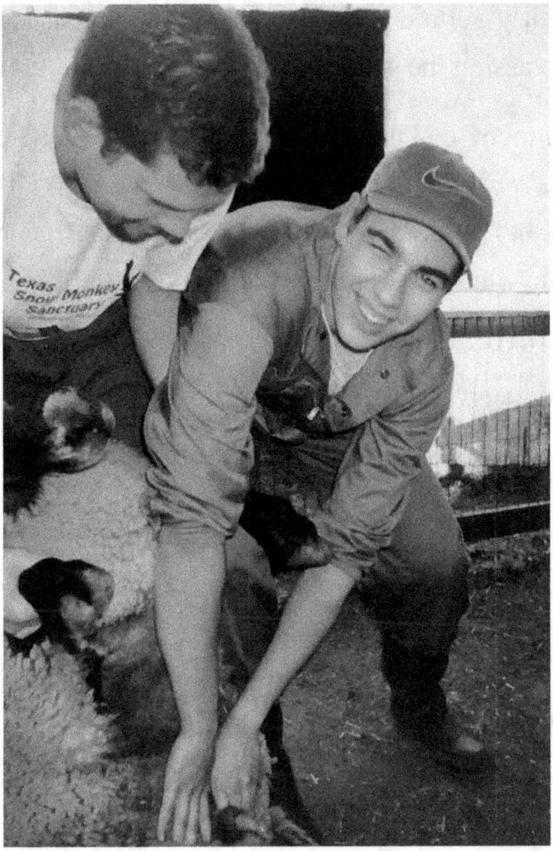

Figure 9. Ram Penis

Chapter 7

My first ever emergency

Emergency medicine doesn't come easily to most medical professionals. It takes a certain type of person to pursue it as a career. During my internship, I wasn't sure I was cut out for it.

In emergency medicine, you're inevitably thrust into high-pressure situations—cases you may or may not have learned about in veterinary school. And often, as a new doctor, without the experience or specialized training to lean on, you're unsure how to proceed. That's not a good feeling, especially when a life is on the line. It's one of the main reasons many veterinarians avoid emergency work altogether.

Yes, they teach us the common emergencies in vet school—gastric dilatation and volvulus (GDV), or "twisted stomach," and ruptured splenic tumors causing internal bleeding, to name a couple. But what they *don't* teach nearly enough about is the human side of veterinary medicine: dealing with the owners. These are family members of the animals we treat, people who are often forced to make heart-wrenching decisions in emotionally charged moments.

They also don't teach you how to handle the moments when you're staring down a case or procedure you've never seen, never practiced, and maybe only read about in a textbook—something you hoped you'd never actually have to deal with. And suddenly, all eyes are on you. You're the doctor now. The pressure is real. The clock is ticking. And you have to make a decision—an educated guess—on how to move forward.

Even now, with years of experience behind me, I still encounter new situations and procedures I've never done before. But now, those moments no longer bring dread—they bring curiosity, and sometimes even a bit of excitement. That's one of the best parts of emergency medicine: no two days are the same, and you never know what's coming through the door.

Back during my internship, though, I felt like I had left every comfort behind. I didn't just leave my childhood home—I left my hometown, my home country, and the safety net of veterinary school, where help was always nearby. I had gone from the small city of Saskatoon, Saskatchewan, all the way to Los Angeles, California, to begin my internship.

I made this move to do an internship—an additional year of practical education that only a small percentage of new veterinarians pursue. They say an internship is like cramming five years of practical experience into one. As a new veterinarian, you're exposed to a wide variety of situations and get the chance to work closely with specialists. It's a year filled with "firsts"—your first laceration repair, your first vomiting dog, even your first diabetic crisis. The advantage is that you have mentors to help guide you through each challenge.

I joined a specialty practice in Los Angeles for my internship. We rotated through several specialty services in the hospital—surgery, internal medicine, oncology, and more. We also had emergency duties. While our emergency department wasn't especially busy, and the emergencies themselves were often routine, we still had hospitalized patients to monitor overnight. Most of the ER cases weren't anything too major, since I was working at a smaller facility, but we definitely didn't have the kind of support system that I now provide to the new doctors at my current hospital.

On my very first ER shift, the phone rang—and panic rang through my bones right along with it. I secretly hoped they wouldn't come in, but of course, the owners did. They were calling about their cat, who had developed a lump on her face that was growing larger and seemed painful. The owners were understandably worried.

Thankfully, my veterinary training kicked in. I took a thorough history and performed a physical exam. Then I sat with the owners for more than 20 minutes, explaining the possible diagnoses: it could be an abscess, feline acne, a tumor—maybe even cancer. The only way to know for sure, I explained, was to start with some bloodwork and to aspirate the mass.

Internally, I was terrified—but fortunately for their pet, the owners agreed to the tests. What they didn't know was that behind my outwardly confident demeanor, I was shaking in my boots.

My mind was racing with "what-ifs." What if it's cancer? What if facial surgery is needed in the middle of the night? What if I get the diagnosis wrong or administer the wrong medication? I had never even used most of the drugs in my ER kit before. What if I messed up the dosage?

Despite all of that, they trusted me with their beloved cat. I administered a light sedative and aspirated the mass. Then I looked at the sample under the microscope, fully aware of the pressure building inside me.

And there it was. The diagnosis was staring right back at me. I saw red blood cells, neutrophils (a type of white blood cell), and then, nestled among the mess, I spotted it: bacteria! Thank goodness—it was an abscess! A simple bacterial infection. A straightforward diagnosis. A curable condition.

I almost sprinted back into the exam room to share the news. I explained to the owners that I had identified the issue, and that it was a good diagnosis—a treatable one. I told them their cat would need antibiotics and some pain relief, but that she should recover just fine.

As I walked out of the room, I was overwhelmed with relief. This had been my first solo case. I'd taken the history, performed the exam, made the diagnosis, communicated the plan—and done it all without backup.

I had done it.That first overnight ER shift continued on without any further emergencies, and I carried that quiet pride with me the rest of the night. I kept replaying the moment in my mind—how I'd been so worried about that cat, unsure of what the mass might be, and how I'd rattled off all the possible (and terrifying) diagnoses to the owners, including cancer. Then, somehow, I'd brought it all back to a simple, treatable abscess. At the time, I was so consumed by fear and adrenaline, I didn't really notice how the owners were feeling.

A few weeks later, I received a letter in the mail from them. I've received similar notes many times since in my career, but this one was my first. It was a letter of thanks.

"Thank you so much for helping our cat. We will never forget your caring hand and the diagnosis you made. What a relief that it was just an infection."

They shared that their cat was doing well, and reading their words filled me with pride all over again.

...but the letter continued.

"Dr. Linklater, I know you're new to the area, and if you'd like to get together for a drink or dinner sometime, please call me." (She included her phone number.)"You are such a sweet person, and I'd love to get to know you better."

It was... a date proposal. From a client.

I wasn't quite sure how to react. I was single at the time, but I also knew that going out with a client wasn't appropriate. Most confusing of all—I had no recollection of what she looked like, how she spoke to me, or anything about her personality. I couldn't even remember exactly who she was. Was it a mother and daughter who brought the cat in? Which one was she? Did she even speak to me at length? I genuinely didn't know.

I'm sure she was a perfectly lovely person—and certainly brave to put herself out there in a handwritten letter (this was back before texting and dating apps were the norm, after all). But I had been so locked into my own fear and anxiety that night that all of the details about the owner just didn't register.

Still, the letter was a kind of ego boost I didn't know I needed. Sometimes encouragement comes from unexpected places—and at exactly the right time. Just a few weeks later, I received some disappointing news: I hadn't been accepted into the ophthalmology residency I had hoped for. I was crushed. I had pinned so many hopes on it, only to be told I "didn't make the cut."

Shortly after that, I spoke to one of my mentors about what to do next. Without hesitation, he suggested I apply for a residency in Emergency and Critical Care. I followed his advice, applied, was accepted—and never looked back.

Emergency medicine is my life now. Although that first emergency didn't lead to a dinner date, it did offer something far more important: a spark. A glimpse into a side of veterinary medicine I hadn't fully imagined for myself. That small moment helped nudge me toward a future that is challenging, unpredictable, and deeply rewarding.

And I couldn't imagine doing anything else.

Chapter 8

My first surgical experience

Medical professionals—or at least most veterinarians—must eventually become comfortable with surgery. Every vet has a first surgical experience. Some are more memorable than others. Mine was certainly memorable, though probably not for the reasons you'd expect.

My "first time" was in veterinary school during a surgical lab that involved sheep. This particular kind of first surgical experience is something that's been phased out at most veterinary schools. Today, the use of live animals for the sole purpose of teaching surgical skills has largely been eliminated. Thanks to technological advancements and improved simulation materials, it's simply no longer necessary. But when I went to vet school, we still used live animals in teaching labs.

Now, for anyone concerned about the animals, please know this: veterinarians—and veterinary students—care deeply for animals. That's part of why these labs have mostly disappeared. But even back then, every effort was made to ensure the animals were treated with respect. They were well-fed, given appropriate medical care, and never allowed to suffer. Faculty coordinated procedures so that each animal could be used in multiple, meaningful ways, always with the animal's well-being in mind.

For this lab, our class was divided into groups of three: a surgeon, an assistant surgeon, and an anesthetist. (We also had a licensed anesthesiologist overseeing the entire process.) I think I drew the short straw—at least that's how I remember it—because I was the primary surgeon in the first round.

We were given instructions the day before, with an emphasis on performing the procedure quickly, precisely, and with as little discomfort to the animal as possible. I studied hard the night before, wanting everything to go perfectly. But despite my preparation, I was riddled with anxiety. It's one of the few moments in my life I can remember feeling physically ill from nerves.

Veterinarians tend to share similar personality traits: we are notoriously hard on ourselves, demand excellence, and expect perfection. There are various moments in our training where we're forced to step into a leadership role—and this was one of them. I would be the one holding the scalpel. I would make the first cut. I would be the one responsible for creating a controlled injury and then stitching everything back together. That responsibility weighed heavily on me.

I didn't sleep at all the night before. I couldn't eat breakfast the next morning. Maybe I'm just looking for excuses, but I think these factors added to the intensity of what I was about to experience.

The sheep were anesthetized and prepped by the anesthesiologist and technician team—people who had done this thousands of times. For them, it was routine. For us, it was brand new. And for me, it was overwhelming.

So, there I was: tired, hungry, and anxious—the perfect trifecta for someone about to perform their very first surgery, right?

To add another layer to the already nerve-wracking situation, we had to fully scrub in for the procedure. Step one: put on a cap and mask. You know—because nothing boosts your confidence like trapping heat on your head and breathing your own hot breath.

Next came the scrub. There's a technique to surgical scrubbing, and although it's evolved over the years, we were trained in the traditional five-minute method with a chlorhexidine scrub brush: one minute on each hand, one minute on each arm, then an extra thirty seconds on each hand again.

Hovering over us was the technician instructor known for her strict adherence to protocol. Honestly, she was a bit terrifying—but in hindsight, she was just doing what was best for the animals. She had a saying: *"If your deltoids don't burn by the end of your scrub, you're not doing it right."* And she wasn't wrong. Keeping your fingertips pointed skyward above your shoulders for five continuous minutes is no small feat. It's necessary, though, so the water flows from your fingers *up* to your elbows, not back down and contaminating the cleanest part—your hands.

After completing the scrub without a misstep, I carefully rinsed, dried off with a sterile towel (in a very specific manner), and began to gown up. You must be extremely cautious during this phase: touch the wrong surface, and you'll contaminate yourself and have to start over from square one.

After donning my gown, I had to spin around to tie it, then push through two doors *with my back* (so as not to use my hands), requiring two more awkward spins. Then came the gloves.

Putting on surgical gloves might look simple, especially if you've only ever seen it done in human hospitals where there's usually an assistant helping you. Not so in vet med. There's no assistant standing by to stretch the glove open for you.

The gloves come folded back at the wrist, and you're only allowed to touch the inside surface. But your hands aren't even *out* of the gown yet! You have to reach into your sleeve, grab the cuff from the inside, then maneuver the glove over your hand—without touching the outside of the glove or your gown. There's a whole choreography to it, and while it becomes second nature with practice, it feels maddeningly awkward the first few times.

And just when you think it can't get more frustrating: no more talc powder to help slide the gloves on. Latex is out, and the newer materials don't always glide easily over damp hands or gowns. It's like trying to fit a wet balloon over another wet balloon—while wearing mittens.

So, to recap: I was tired, hungry, anxious, hot, sweaty, sore, dizzy, *and* frustrated from trying to get those gloves on. A less-than-ideal combination going into your first live surgery. Then, just as I stepped up to the table, all the wrong memories started creeping in—like the first time I smelled burning flesh, or my visit to the hot dog factory. Oh yes, that smell. My body didn't love the recall.

Anxious, sleep-deprived, hungry (or maybe borderline malnourished), sore, dizzy, nauseated, and completely stressed. It was vet school, after all, and no one liked being first. Guess who was first? Me. Just another layer of pressure.

Still, I managed to step up to the sheep on the table. I began draping the surgical field with sterile cloths, trying to focus, though a cold sweat had already broken out across my back. I placed the scalpel blade onto the handle and turned to the anesthetist for confirmation that everything was ready. I got *the nod.*

There's a photo of me in the large animal surgical bay from that day (Figure 10). You can't tell from the distance, but I was definitely *not* feeling okay. That bay, in retrospect, looked more like something out of an old-timey surgery scene from *MASH** than a modern operating suite. But that's where it all started.My first incision—a simple straight line through the skin. *"Okay, so far,"* I told myself. The second cut through the subcutaneous tissue. Then came the final slice through the midline body wall—muscle and fascia. There was some blood, but not too much.

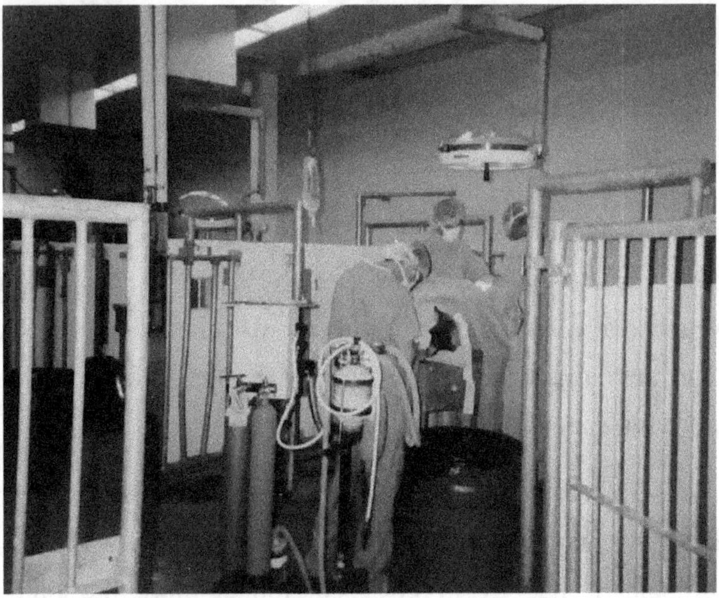

Figure 10. Hot Ass Surgery

I was doing fine… up until then.

No one had quite prepared me for what it feels like—the smell, the texture—when you're holding the inside of a living animal. The organs are hot, wet, and slick. And when a loop of intestine slid out and landed in my hand, I froze. I was suddenly holding the vital, beating, bloody insides of a breathing sheep—and the cold sweat hit me like a wave. My head started spinning.

I could actually *feel* the blood drain from my face. My lips went numb. I realized then exactly why a surgical assistant exists. I'd been in this position before (as you've read earlier)… but never quite like this.

Spots danced in my vision.

Let's take inventory again: anxious, sleep-deprived, probably hypoglycemic, sore, overheated, dizzy, nauseated, stressed. The perfect storm.

Before the lab began, the instructors had warned us not to be embarrassed if we had to scrub out of surgery. It apparently happened every year. "About 10–15% of students," they said. "Some pass out. Some vomit. That's why we have backup." They reassured us that this was the time to make mistakes—while surrounded by support. "Your assistant is here to take over if needed." Everyone always thinks, *that won't be me.*

Until it is.

I suppose I was lucky—I recognized the signs. Still holding the warm, slippery intestines of a sheep, I raised my hand, careful not to contaminate anything. My hand didn't go very high—I was too lightheaded for that—and I quietly said I needed to sit down.

"We've got our first!" my instructor called out.

"What?!" I muttered in disbelief, as I was quickly surrounded by technicians who gently ushered me out of the suite and into a side room. They sat me down, took off my gown, placed a cool cloth on my neck, and had me bend forward to keep from fainting.

Thankfully, I never actually passed out. But I came close.

My group stepped in and finished the procedure without me. And just as I started to collect myself, I heard a crash from the surgical suite. One of my classmates had gone down—flat on the floor. She hadn't seen the warning signs and tried to power through. She didn't make it.

As much as I felt embarrassed, I was grateful I wasn't *her*.

The instructors and my teammates were incredibly supportive. "Don't worry about it," they said. "You were first. All the pressure was on you. And hey—you didn't hit the floor!"

Still, I learned something important about myself that day. And I wasn't alone—misery really does love company.

Ironically, these days, I handle some of the most critical trauma cases and complicated surgeries of my career, and none of it fazes me. I've come a long way from that first sheep surgery, and now I get to pass that story on to new interns when they feel faint or overwhelmed in the OR. It's one of my favorites to tell—because it reminds me how far I've come, and how we *all* start somewhere.

Chapter 9

The Second Largest Volume of Blood I Have Ever Seen

This story takes place during my final year of veterinary school. I was an eager beaver—determined to impress my professors. By this point, I already knew I was heading into a small animal rotating internship, but we had chosen our fourth-year rotations more than a year prior. Despite my focus on small animals, the curriculum required a minimum number of large animal rotations. So, like many of my classmates, I had to strategically choose how to meet that requirement.

Naturally, I scheduled my large animal rotations in the fall or spring—anything to avoid those brutally cold Saskatchewan winters. I had endured enough of them by that point.

For this particular rotation, I selected an ambulatory equine course, meaning we would leave campus in one of the school's mobile veterinary trucks to visit farms, stables, or racetracks. We'd perform various procedures on-site—anything from vaccinations and dental work to lameness exams. Most of the places we visited had scheduled appointments in advance, but occasionally, we'd respond to emergency calls.

As fate would have it, this day turned out to be a good one. It was late spring in Saskatchewan—finally, some warmth and sunshine after the long winter. Even better, calving season had just ended, so we weren't expecting to be elbow-deep in any difficult births. And since I was on the equine rotation, I had another stroke of luck: most of the animals we saw were well cared for.

Just for context—this isn't always the case with large animals. Horses, often considered companion animals, tend to receive a higher standard of care. Cattle, on the other hand, are typically seen as production animals, and unfortunately, their medical care is sometimes dictated more by economics than compassion. If the cost of treatment exceeds the animal's value, care is often declined. It's a hard truth many of us learned early on.Anyway, it was the final day of our equine rotation. Two eager vet students—myself included—were riding in the truck with our clinician, enjoying the prospect of wrapping up the week. That's when the radio crackled to life.

"Hi there, folks," came the voice over the pager system that linked all ambulatory units. "We just received a call from a local farmer located about 45 to 50 minutes from your current location. He's got a cow in the paddock that's giving birth and having a major issue. He suspects a prolapse and needs someone to come out right away."

A prolapse. That's a real emergency. Any time internal organs are outside the body, it's critical and time-sensitive.

But we were on an equine rotation. Surely this wasn't our call to take. We exchanged a quick glance, silently willing one of the bovine ambulatory units to answer the emergency call. It was 4 p.m. on a beautiful Friday afternoon—our last day on this rotation—and neither of us was on call. We were so close to being done. We could almost taste the weekend.

Then, silence.

The radio stayed quiet far too long, the kind of long that makes your stomach sink. We kept driving toward the vet college, inching closer to freedom, when the radio buzzed again.

"Hi again. I see car #7 on the equine rotation had a light day and should be heading back by now. I've paged the bovine ambulatory units, but no one's responded. I know you're the equine group, but could you check out this cow?"

Our clinician sighed. I'm pretty sure we all shared the same internal monologue. But she picked up the radio and answered, "OK, we'll go check it out."

We shot her a look that said, *Seriously?* She chuckled and apologized, "Sorry, guys! Hopefully we can just take a quick look, make a recommendation, and be on our way. If it's as serious as the farmer says, he'll likely need to bring the cow to the college for surgery." The equine service trucks are not equipped for full anesthesia—maybe sedation and minor procedures, but not major surgery.

That gave us some hope. Maybe this was just a quick stop. Maybe we'd still make it back home or at least to the veterinary college before the sun went down.So, after a 45-minute drive, we arrived at the farm. The local farmer waved us toward the correct paddock. It was a medium-sized enclosure—maybe half an acre—with a dozen cows milling about. One stood out immediately, isolated from the rest.

This was a dairy farm, and the cow in question was a big Holstein—the familiar black-and-white breed you see on milk cartons and in TV ads. From a distance, we could see she was lying down in the grass, and something large and pink was protruding from her back end.

The farmer approached and explained, "She's been trying to deliver a calf most of the day. I wasn't sure if it was stuck or sideways or something. I tried pulling, but then all this tissue just started coming out."

We opened the gate and walked toward her. She didn't move. She was down.

Now, for context—when a large animal is "down," it's a serious problem. In terms of trying to move a down cow, three relatively small humans, even with our combined strength are no match for a 1,500 to 2,000-pound cow. And when cows lie down too long, especially during calving, they can compress major nerves and blood vessels in their hind limbs. Unlike us, they can't just "shake it off." Once circulation is compromised, they physically *can't* stand. We call this a "down cow," and it's always concerning.

We tried everything—coaxing, pulling, pushing, even a few well-intentioned slaps to the rear. Nothing. She was completely exhausted.

And then we got a closer look.

Her uterus had prolapsed. Completely. In her effort to deliver the calf, she had pushed her entire uterus out through her birth canal. A massive, bulbous mass—easily over a hundred pounds—hung from her hind end. The exposed tissue was drying out, dirty, and already showing signs of damage from lost blood flow.

We started by lavaging the tissue—flushing it clean with sterile fluids—and tried to remove the calf manually. We also attempted to reposition and push the uterus back in, but with her lying down and not moving, there was no leverage. No cooperation from her body. It wasn't working.

At that point, the decision had to be made. And by "we," I mean the clinician—because I was still a student, and frankly, I had no idea what I was doing beyond following instructions. She told the farmer the only viable option was to get the cow onto a trailer and bring her back to the veterinary school for surgery.

Reluctantly, the farmer agreed.

Now comes the scary part.

The farmer had to go get his truck and trailer, as we did not come with a trailer. Luckily (or so I thought) the paddock was large enough to drive his truck into, right up beside the cow. This was going to immensely help our efforts to get the cow loaded up for transport. We could even use the truck to help her get up, if we could line things up just right.

So, the farmer left the paddock and walked around to hook up his old trailer—rusty, loud, and barely holding itself together. He moved the truck toward us, and we opened the paddock gate, doing our best to keep the other curious cows from wandering out.

And wouldn't you know it? The cow could walk after all—or at least, she tried.

Startled by the truck and trailer pulling up beside her, she gave it a go. We were momentarily relieved—if she could stand, maybe we had a fighting chance of loading her up without needing ropes or pulleys. But her legs, numb from hours of lying on one side, betrayed her. Our hopes of getting her loaded up successfully were quickly dashed by what happened next.

She staggered forward, took two unstable steps, and then fell—hard.

And she didn't just fall anywhere—she fell right onto the sharp, jagged corner of the trailer's side panel. The metal edge sliced into her like a blade. We gasped as we saw the wound—a massive gash, easily two feet long and six inches deep, slashing right through the most swollen, vascular part of her prolapsed uterus.

It was as if someone had opened a fire hydrant of blood.

The vessels torn in the process weren't just small capillaries—they were thick, engorged uterine arteries and veins, the size of pencils... even sausages. (A comparison I've come to appreciate more after living in Wisconsin for years—where bratwurst is practically its own food group.)

The bleeding was immediate and catastrophic.

I have only seen that much blood one other time in my life—and this was right up there. With each heartbeat, more blood sprayed from the torn vessels. In seconds, we were ankle-deep in it. The ground beneath us turned into a crimson pond, easily eight feet wide and growing by the second.

Instinct and training kicked in. The three of us leapt into action, trying to grab hold of the gaping wound, putting pressure on vessels, trying desperately to stem the flow. We slowed it a little—but not enough. Not nearly enough.

Within a minute, it was clear: she was bleeding out. Fast.

We had no time, no options. The only decision left to make was the hardest one. We couldn't save her. But maybe—just maybe—we could save the calf.

The call was made: sacrifice the mother to try and save the baby.

Now, here's what most people don't realize about farm animal euthanasia. When you're dealing with a food animal like a cow, you can't just give her a chemical euthanasia injection like we would in companion animals—it renders the meat unsafe and unfit for any use. And in cases like this, that's still a financial and emotional disaster for the farmer (moreso than what was already happening).

So the standard, humane option for emergency euthanasia on-farm is to shoot the animal—a single, carefully aimed shot to the head, ending life instantly.

But here's the kicker: we were on the *equine* service. And the equine service didn't carry a gun.

Only the bovine unit carried guns—and they were nowhere nearby.

That left us with two options, neither good: give her a lethal injection and render the body unusable, or find a firearm immediately.

We turned to the farmer and asked, "Do you have a gun?"

He nodded and rushed off to fetch it while we stayed behind, preparing the cow and clearing the area. Even in a moment like this, training matters. Knowing how to shoot an animal humanely and effectively is something we're taught in veterinary school. It's not just about ending suffering—it's about doing it *right.*

We prepared. In your mind's eye, you draw an imaginary 'X' across the animal's forehead—one line from the right eye to the left ear, and the other from the left eye to the right ear. Where those lines cross, just above the center of the eyes, is the target. That's where the shot needs to go. The site is a little higher than most people would expect. And if you miss, you instead have a cow in more pain with a very bloody nose (I have seen it done incorrectly).

It's a grim task. But in moments like this, grim tasks are the only humane ones left.

The clinician spent a minute reviewing the procedure with us—how to position the shot, what to expect, and how quickly we'd need to work afterward. While we stood in the growing puddle of blood, trying to mentally prepare, the farmer headed off to retrieve his gun.

A few minutes later, he returned... rifle slung casually over his forearm, loading bullets into the chamber as he strolled back toward us—like it was just another day at the park. Then, with a loud *click*, he cocked the gun mid-stride and—unbelievably—continued sauntering toward us, muzzle swinging freely, pointing right at all three of us.

I lost it, "Point that *f**ing** thing at the ground! Are you trying to kill us?!" I yelled.

That was probably one of the only times I've sworn openly in front of an instructor. But at that moment, I really didn't care. I didn't go through all those years of school to die in a cow paddock at the hands of Farmer McTrigger Happy. My sudden outburst stunned everyone—the farmer froze, the other student blinked, and even the clinician's jaw dropped. Not exactly the image of professional composure I usually tried to uphold... but I stand by my comments to this day!

The farmer, looking sheepish, realized what he'd done and quickly pointed the rifle toward the ground. "Sorry, sorry," he mumbled. We walked him through where to aim—just above the center of the eyes, right where the imaginary X intersects. A single, clean shot. Quick and humane.

Then we got ready.

We suited up with gloves and protective gear, knives in hand. The pool of blood had more than doubled now, and everything—ground, hooves, our boots—was slick. We knew the moment the cow was down, it would be go-time.

"Ready?" the clinician asked.

"Ready."

BANG!

The rifle cracked. The cow collapsed. A perfect shot.

Without hesitation, we lunged in.

It wasn't exactly "hack and slash," but it was close. The clinician gave us direction, but our hands were flying. We cut swiftly into the side, through skin, muscle, fat, and into the belly cavity, lifting organs, navigating slick surfaces, making room to reach the swollen uterus. It was like fighting through a living, bleeding obstacle course.

The uterus was massive, still partly prolapsed and soaked with blood. We opened it wide with long, rapid strokes of the scalpel. Blood and amniotic fluid splashed everywhere—covering our arms, faces, chests. I had never been so soaked in my life. Only once more in my career have I had to change clothes top to bottom like that.

Then came the heaving. The calf was easily over 100 pounds—wet, heavy, and so slick with fluid it felt like trying to wrestle a greased water balloon out of a fire hose. We reached in, gently navigating around limbs and the umbilical cord, careful not to cause harm.

And finally—we had him.

We pulled him free, laid him out, and immediately got to work stimulating him. Rubbing, swinging, clearing airways. After a few tense seconds, he gave a gasp, then a cough. His chest rose, then fell.

Then it did so again.

Then a cry.

He was alive!

We all exhaled in near disbelief.

A few minutes later, that calf—blood-covered and shivering—staggered to his feet. It was one of those surreal moments: standing in a literal lake of blood, steam rising from the fresh body nearby, and a newborn calf blinking up at us, alive because we acted fast. For a moment, it reminded me of the birthing of Billy Crystal's cow 'Norman' from the movie City Slickers (the mother of that cow also, didn't make it, thanks to the quick reactions of Jack Palance's character). This version had a lot more blood, however.

It wasn't the ending we had hoped for. We lost the mother. But in the context of veterinary medicine—especially rural, large animal work—sometimes you don't get to choose a perfect outcome. Sometimes you choose *the only* outcome.

And the farmer? He was shaken, but grateful. "Didn't think we'd save the baby," he said, brushing a sleeve across his face. "Thank you."

We cleaned up what we could. Packed our tools, peeled off our dripping gear, and climbed into the truck. Our coveralls were completely soaked. The smell stuck to our skin for days.

As we pulled away, I looked back at the paddock. That crimson lake, the quiet animals, the calf wobbling toward the water trough.

You never forget moments like that. Not the blood. Not the chaos. Not the adrenaline. And definitely not the reminder that, in veterinary medicine, you don't just treat animals—you make hard, fast, human decisions in the middle of messy, unpredictable realities.

That was a rough day…obviously stuck with me. I *did* earn a new kind of respect—for life, for death, and for just how damn fast things can change.

Section 2

I Can't Believe You Ate The Whole Thing!

Chapter 1

Introduction

This chapter is mostly about the things animals get into—and eat—but I can't begin those stories without a brief introduction to the food culture inside veterinary hospitals, especially 24-hour facilities.

Regulations laid out by the Occupational Safety and Health Administration (OSHA) clearly specify where food intended for human consumption can be kept in a veterinary hospital. That said, these rules are often ignored—especially in busy settings and particularly when "the boss" (whoever that may be) isn't around. Cups filled with beverages and various snacks can regularly be found sitting on counters or tucked away in pockets.

There's always a risk in a veterinary hospital of forgetting that your snack or drink is in your pocket—or worse, on the counter. Every so often, someone's food or drink ends up sitting alarmingly close to something disgusting… or something disgusting ends up in a pocket. There's a reason OSHA put those regulations in place: not just to keep things sanitary, but also to minimize health risks. Food and drink left near animals—especially those carrying infectious diseases—can pose a real danger.

Still, in the chaos of a workday, when someone yells for help from across the treatment room or you're returning from a break, it's easy to set your drink on the nearest counter without thinking. When you're rushing to assist with a procedure, OSHA protocols sometimes fall by the wayside.

I've even managed to snap a few photos of these all-too-common situations. Figure 1, for example, shows a glass of (presumably) lemonade sitting next to a large bowl of bloody fluid. It really makes you think: would you still want to drink that lemonade? What are the chances something splashed into it? These liquids are way too close for comfort—could there have been some cross-contamination? Or, even worse, is that really lemonade... or something else entirely?

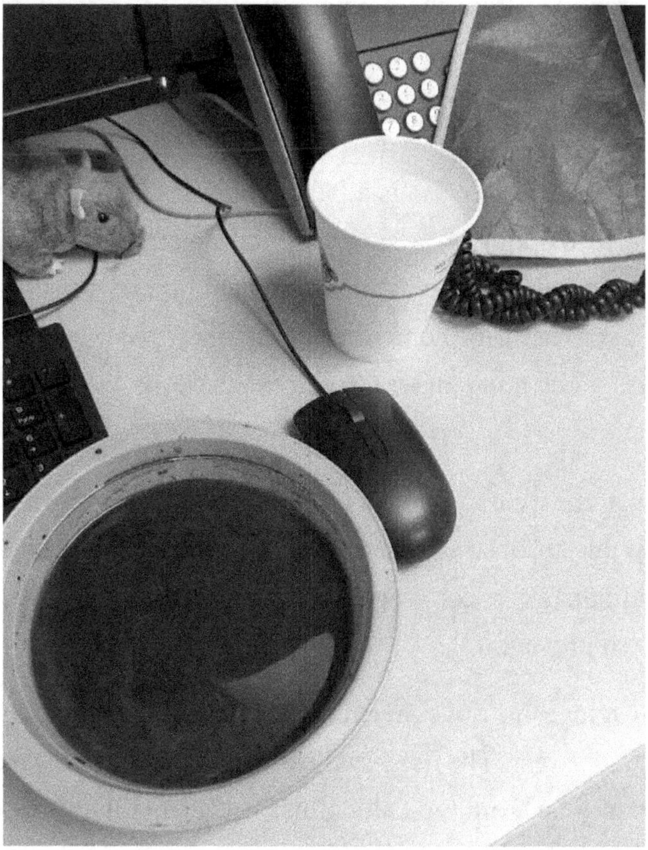

Figure 1

How risky are you willing to be when it comes to drinking that "lemonade"? And how thirsty are you, really? If it were your cup and you were the one who left it there, I'd bet that most of the time, that lemonade would still get consumed. I do my best to enforce the rules around the hospital, but believe me, I've seen far worse.

At one veterinary clinic I visited, there was an open birthday cake—store-bought and uncovered—sitting right next to the table where a dental procedure was underway. That made me feel a little sick. During dental procedures, all kinds of material are constantly being propelled from the animal's mouth. I'd be willing to bet that something from the dog's mouth ended up in that cake.

Crunch.

Anyway, this section is all about animals getting into things they shouldn't. Working in a small animal emergency room, I've seen countless cases where pets have ingested objects or substances they weren't supposed to. Sometimes, what they swallow turns out to be harmless—but other times, it can be toxic or lead to an intestinal obstruction.

Over the years, I've had to take two of my own dogs in for surgery due to obstructions caused by things they'd ingested. So I know firsthand: it can happen, even when you try your absolute hardest to prevent it.

Most ingestions we see are pretty routine—chocolate, marijuana, socks, underwear. The list is endless. But every so often, a case comes along that's far from typical—either because of the sheer quantity of what was eaten, the bizarre nature of the item, or a completely unexpected twist in the story. Sometimes animals ingest more than one thing at once, which adds an extra layer of chaos. It's particularly amusing when a dog comes in for eating one thing… and you discover so much more inside!

Several of those memorable cases are coming up.

I lecture at veterinary conferences regularly, and toxins are one of my favorite topics to cover. Part of the reason is that I didn't feel I mastered toxicology particularly well during vet school—but working in emergency medicine has forced me to become an expert. And now that I truly understand it, I find toxicology fascinating.

The nuances of working with toxins are immense. Sometimes it's hard to keep them all straight. For example: did you know there are multiple classes of rodenticides (rat and mouse poisons)? In fact, there are dozens upon dozens of individual toxins that fall under that general category—and each one may require a different treatment protocol.

There are several steps we follow at the veterinary hospital when an animal eats something that isn't pet food—and yes, even some human foods can be toxic to dogs and cats. First, we determine whether the substance ingested is potentially toxic. If it is, the next question is: did the animal ingest enough to cause clinical signs of toxicity—or worse, death?

We also have to consider whether the ingested item could result in an intestinal obstruction, perforation, ulcers, or other serious complications. These assessments guide us in deciding how and when to intervene.

If intervention is necessary, our first question is often whether we can decontaminate the animal by inducing emesis (vomiting). This is commonly done with an injectable medication, which tends to work quite reliably in dogs—though much less so in cats.

If the toxin is one that could still be absorbed from the gastrointestinal tract, we may follow the emesis with activated charcoal, administered orally, to bind any remaining toxin in the stomach. However, inducing vomiting isn't always safe or effective. So we must ask ourselves a series of critical questions—each one requiring clinical judgment based on the specifics of the case. Here are a few of the main ones, along with examples from real-life scenarios:

1. **Which toxins are safe to induce vomiting for?**
   Some toxins, particularly corrosive substances, can cause burns to the esophagus and stomach. In these cases, vomiting may do more harm than good.
   Example: Pool chemicals.

2. **Was something sharp ingested?**
   Sharp objects can perforate the stomach or damage the throat during vomiting.
   Examples: Needles, fish hooks, even knives.

3. **Is it safe to induce vomiting in this particular patient?**
   Certain health conditions may increase the risk of aspiration pneumonia if vomiting is induced.
   Example: Brachycephalic breeds like Pugs and French Bulldogs are especially prone to aspiration.

4. **Will inducing vomiting be effective?**
   If too much time has passed, the stomach may have already emptied. Additionally, large or obstructive items often don't come up through emesis.
   Examples: Tennis balls, bones, or esophageal obstructions.

5. **What dose of the toxin was ingested?**
   We do our best to calculate this based on available information, but often details are unclear—like how much medication was left in a bottle. Sometimes, the dose isn't lethal, but when in doubt, we assume the worst and monitor the animal closely.
   Example: Marijuana toxicity can take hours to manifest; with substances like grapes, raisins, or rat poison, signs may not appear for several days.

6. **Is it safe and effective to administer charcoal?**
   Not all toxins bind to charcoal. And if the patient is too sedated, it may not be safe to administer it orally.
   Example: Antifreeze is rapidly absorbed, causes sedation, and doesn't bind to charcoal.

7. **Which toxins are eliminated by the kidneys or could damage them?**
   In such cases, aggressive fluid therapy may be required, including IV fluids and hospitalization.
   Example: Lilies are extremely toxic to cats, and fluids are always recommended.

8. **Which toxins have immediate effects, and which take time?** Many toxins won't cause symptoms right away. That's why early decontamination is always preferred to dealing with consequences days later.
Examples: Vitamin D, antifreeze, anticoagulant rodenticides.

The bottom line is this: treating toxic or foreign-body ingestion isn't as simple as "pumping the stomach and sending the pet home." There are countless nuances, and each case is a little different.

So let's meander through some of the more interesting ingestions I've seen over the years, shall we?

Chapter 2

Jack and his Frequent Flyer Card

Jack the Labrador Retriever was a little… well, different. He was a very friendly young black Lab, and we saw Jack at the hospital again and again for his unique ingestions. You can even see him licking his lips in the picture—a very cute and lovable dog (Figure 2). But Jack had a bad habit: he loved eating things he wasn't supposed to.

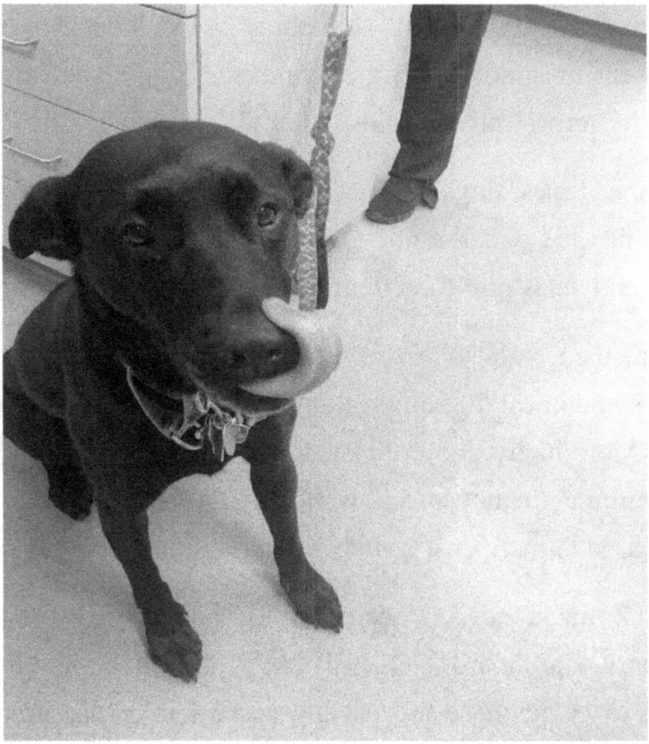

Figure 2. Jack

This kind of behavior isn't exactly rare in young Labradors, as many of you probably know. Jack, however, had developed a particular taste. Luckily, it wasn't something toxic—but it *was* something that could potentially cause an obstruction: cardboard. Jack ate a *lot* of cardboard. And he did it *frequently*.

Sometimes, animals develop habits like this due to behavioral issues, such as separation anxiety. Other times, it might be related to a medical condition. For instance, it's well documented that animals with anemia (low red blood cell count) may eat unusual things like dirt or metal. Pets with nutritional deficiencies or absorption issues may do the same. And occasionally, a pet simply develops a taste for a particular item—often something we'd consider gross, like underwear or condoms. But remember: a dog's standards for what counts as "gross" are *very* low. After all, they do lick their own butts.

Other times, dogs are just being silly. They don't know what's digestible and what's not—they're ridiculous. When an animal consistently eats non-food items, we refer to that behavior as **pica**.

But then… there are *Labradors*. Labradors are just a *little* bit dumb sometimes! I shouldn't say "dumb," actually—they're quite smart. More likely, they're just a little bored. They start chewing on things around the house, and while it might taste awful to us, it either tastes good to them or it's simply entertaining.

Jack made several visits to us, and most were for eating cardboard. Cardboard itself isn't toxic—though it may have glue or adhesives on it, those are usually present in small, non-dangerous amounts. What we *do* worry about is the cardboard balling up in the intestines and causing an obstruction. That's a real risk. We always had to ask if there was anything inside the cardboard that Jack ate—just to make sure there wasn't a toxic substance hiding inside. Luckily for Jack, it was always just the cardboard.

The good news? It's fairly easy to make dogs vomit. We use an injectable medication called **apomorphine**, and it works more than 90% of the time. So, after each ingestion, once we assessed how much Jack had eaten—and whether it was chewed into small pieces—we'd induce vomiting. If we recovered enough cardboard, and Jack was stable, we sent him home almost immediately.

Jack started this habit at five years old, and no one really knows why. Sometimes the cardboard had something tasty in it (like a loaf of bread); other times, there was nothing at all. Maybe he was bored. Maybe he was hungry. Or maybe—most likely—Jack was just being a Labrador.

As the weeks went by (and it took some time to realize this), we noticed that Jack was coming in about once a month after eating something he shouldn't have—and more often than not, it was cardboard. His owners were fantastic—always prioritizing Jack's health, even with his frustrating little habit. After his third visit, they authorized a full workup, including bloodwork and X-rays, to rule out any medical conditions that might be causing the behavior.

By Jack's fifth visit, we decided to have a little fun with the situation. We made Jack a **"Frequent Vomiter Card"** (Figure 3). Not exactly a badge of honor, but it was our way of injecting some humor into the ordeal. It was basically a punch card: "Buy nine trips to the vet for vomiting induction, and the tenth one is free." Each visit was initialed by the attending veterinarian, and when I took the photo, Jack had already reached episode number four.

This obviously isn't something veterinary hospitals do every day—but for us, it lightened the mood, and Jack's owner appreciated the gesture.

We even threw in a little twist: the card was *made out of cardboard*—Jack's favorite foreign material. Maybe it was a fail-safe… or maybe we just have a twisted sense of humor.

I never did find out if Jack made it to that tenth free visit.

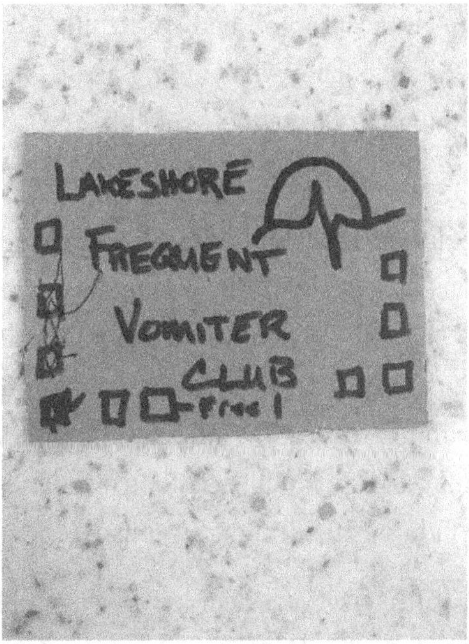

Figure 3. The Frequent Vomiter

Chapter 3

Why the heck are you eating all that grass?

We're often left wondering why animals eat the strange things they do. What was the motivation? Did that object really smell or taste good enough to eat? These days, my usual response is: their standards are pretty low. As I mentioned earlier—they lick their own butts. So, let's temper our expectations.

One of the most common questions we get is: *"Why is my dog eating grass?"* People are constantly puzzled by this behavior. But the answer isn't actually that mysterious, nor is it beyond the reach of science. In fact, it's quite simple: grass serves a variety of purposes for dogs.

Think about it—plenty of animals derive almost all of their nutrition from plants: cows, goats, bison, deer, rabbits, wildebeest, and so on. Technically, they eat plants to feed the bacteria in their gut, and then they digest those bacteria. It's a brilliant symbiotic system.

So, what about dogs? Dogs don't break down grass the way herbivores do, so why do they eat it?

There are several reasons.

Reason #1: Grass is everywhere.

Even in the modern world, grass is abundant. It grows on nearly every continent (well… maybe not Antarctica), and in North America, we actually *cultivate* it. We water it, fertilize it, and compare our lawns to the neighbors'. Grass is everywhere—we play on it, lie on it, relax in it. So, is it really that surprising that dogs might occasionally nibble on it? Dogs get bored, and sometimes, chewing on grass is just something to pass the time.

Reason #2: Dogs are weird… and kind of gross.

Remember, these are animals that regularly groom themselves by licking their genitals, their butts, their wounds, their feet—and then go straight to licking your face. Compared to that, grass doesn't seem all that bad. But maybe what attracts them isn't just the grass—it's the *stuff* on the grass.

Even in quiet neighborhoods, plenty of wildlife roam through yards: birds, squirrels, cats, rabbits, deer, and of course, other dogs. And with all of them come smells—urine, feces, saliva, vomit, and (a fan favorite for dogs) anal gland secretions. Dogs are natural explorers, and with their noses constantly to the ground, they're just becoming familiar with their environment.

And hey—let's be honest. Most of us have, at some point, put a piece of grass in our mouth as kids. Grass doesn't really taste that bad—it's bland, sure, but not exactly offensive. Some dogs might simply stumble across a bonus snack. I know one of my dogs *loves* to graze on deer and rabbit poop from the yard. Gross, I know… but apparently delicious.

Reason #3: Dogs are bored.

Sometimes, it's just something to do. Nibbling on little green stems can entertain them for hours. I've owned several dogs over the years, and most of them have enjoyed lounging outside, casually chewing on grass like it's their favorite hobby.

Reason #4: Dogs get tummy aches too.

This might be the most important reason of all. For generations, humans have had ways to treat gastrointestinal discomfort. It started with spoonfuls of baking soda. Later, someone got creative and mixed bicarbonate with calcium, added a little sugar, and invented Tums®. Then came the acid blockers—Pepcid, Zantac, Tagamet, omeprazole (Prilosec), lansoprazole, and more. Today, these medications are cheap, widely available, and effective.

Dogs? They don't have a pharmacy. They've got dirt and grass.

So maybe, when a dog's stomach is feeling a bit off, chewing on some grass adds a little bulk and fiber—something that helps settle the gut. Maybe it's instinctual. Maybe it's soothing.

Or maybe, like so many things dogs do… it's just one of their quirks.Makes sense, right? It's not a terribly complicated solution.

However, with grass—as with anything else—too much of a good thing is never good. We certainly don't want our pups eating grass constantly, especially without supervision or limits. Over the years, I've seen a few dogs that ingested excessive amounts—wads and wads and wads of grass—and let me tell you, that's not good.

When a dog consumes large quantities of grass, it can become tangled and compacted in the stomach, leading to gastrointestinal upset, vomiting, and in more severe cases, even significant weight loss.

I've included a picture to illustrate just such a case. We once had a skinny two-year-old female pit bull abandoned at our hospital. She was the sweetest dog, but her previous owners suspected something was wrong. Every time she ate more than half a cup of food, she would vomit it back up.

We took a radiograph (x-ray) of her abdomen, and her stomach appeared full of... something. It was hard to determine exactly what—maybe food, maybe cloth, or possibly even grass. If it was food, it should've passed with time. So, we waited a few hours and took another radiograph. But her stomach remained full.

To get a better view, we administered barium—a contrast agent that outlines the inside of the gastrointestinal tract. (See attached image, Figure 4.) In the x-ray, she's lying on her back, and you can clearly see her enlarged stomach filled with material and barium. Yet, the size of the stomach didn't decrease.

There wasn't an intestinal obstruction, as the barium was making its way through all the loops of her intestines. That led us to conclude she had a chronic foreign object in her stomach.

At that point, the next step was clear: surgery.

Once in the OR, we discovered her stomach was completely packed with grass—matted and compacted into dense wads. It took quite a while to remove it all. This condition is common enough that it even has a name: **phytobezoar**—which essentially means "a plant-based rock." It's a large mass of indigestible plant material, usually stuck in the stomach or elsewhere in the GI tract, preventing normal digestion and absorption.

Fortunately, we had identified the issue. We surgically removed the mass, sutured her stomach closed, and gave her time to recover. The result? This sweet little pit bull bounced back beautifully. No more vomiting. She began eating normally and quickly gained weight.

Best of all, she ended up in a loving forever home—adopted by one of our very own doctors. She's still doing great to this day.

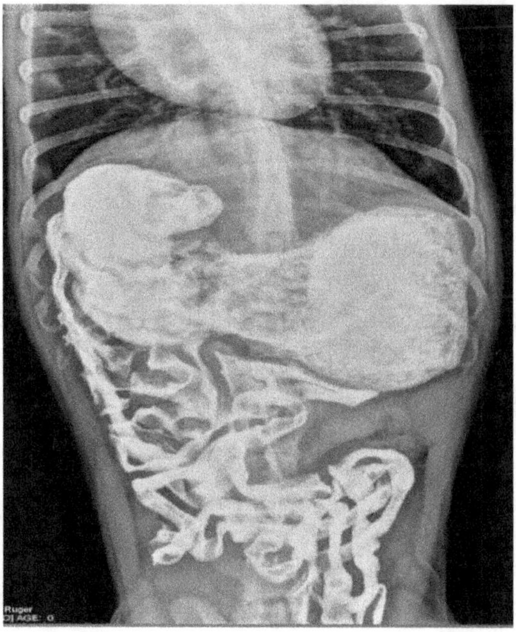

Figure 4.

Chapter 4

Well, we weren't expecting that

Sometimes dogs like to eat delicious things that we also enjoy — peanut butter, for example. Peanut butter is usually great for dogs, they enjoy the taste, it's a great treat and it's also used as a clever tool….a way to hide medications! Cheese works just as well—brick, fake, or cream cheese—all the same. Delicious for us and generally safe for our pets. I'm sure many of you have tried giving your dog peanut butter as a treat, as a way to administer pills, or simply for the entertainment of watching them lick their lips and the roof of their mouth for what seems like 20 minutes. It's great, isn't it? Safe, tasty, nutritious, and it makes those pills go down "lickety-split!" The only downside we usually mention is the calorie content, so you do need to be mindful of how much and how often they get it.

These days, instead of peanut butter, I've switched to canned dog food. It's a little less expensive and lower in calories. However, canned food doesn't stick together as well as peanut butter, so I'm more likely to get my hands involved to make a little ball with the pill inside. Gross, I know—but hey, I do wash afterwards. I've also fed my dogs some vegetables and ice cubes—they think those are treats, too, and they're much better calorie-wise, but not so great for hiding medications!

Well, as it turns out, there are other downsides to peanut butter besides just calories.

Sometimes, we need to be careful *how* we deliver peanut butter - covered pills to dogs. To lead into this next story, think about the last time you gave your dog peanut butter: how did you get the peanut butter out of the jar? A knife or a spoon? It probably depends on what you're using it for, right? If you're a guy grabbing a quick snack, you might just use a spoon. If you're making a sandwich, you probably use a knife. Maybe you're scraping the bottom of the jar with a spatula.

Now imagine scooping peanut butter from the bottom of the jar *to give your dog some pills*. What utensil would you use? Like most of you, I'd probably reach for a spoon.

One day, an innocent owner brought their Great Dane to us after the dog ate something unusual. This dog had recently had a urinary tract infection and was on antibiotics. Of course, antibiotics don't taste great, so the owners used the classic trick: scooping peanut butter from the jar with a spoon, then squishing the capsules into the peanut butter on the spoon, and letting the dog lick it off. It worked perfectly every time. Except one day, it worked a little *too* well.

While giving the medication and peanut butter, the dog *ate and swallowed the whole spoon*! Yes—the entire spoon.

We took an x-ray, and this was one of the rare times where a foreign object was easily identified on the radiograph. Check out the picture in Figure 5! You can clearly see the metal end of the spoon in the dog's stomach. It's worth noting how clearly the metal shows up, while the plastic handle does not. This is a common problem with many foreign objects—they often don't show up well on x-rays.

Nice for us, nice for the dog, nice for the family: problem identified, confirmed, and ready for a solution.

Our options were to remove the spoon with an endoscopy or go to surgery. Inducing vomiting wouldn't likely work because of the spoon's size. The choice was clear: endoscopy is less invasive, less expensive, and offers faster recovery. The owners agreed, and we forged ahead.

We placed an IV catheter to administer injectable anesthesia and inserted an endotracheal tube to provide inhaled anesthesia and protect her airway while we worked. The Great Dane tolerated anesthesia well, and we closely monitored her vital signs.

Using a long (1.5-meter, nearly 5-foot!) flexible scope, we passed it down her mouth, through the esophagus, and into the stomach. We quickly located the spoon, passed a grasping instrument through the scope, grabbed it, and removed the spoon. Success!

But there was more. While assessing the stomach with the scope, we spotted some other colored material. "What's this?" we wondered. The owners hadn't reported anything else missing.

We managed to grasp the material, but it took some effort to pull it out through the esophagus and mouth. After some work, out it came: a sock!

We went back in and found more colored material—another sock. And then another. And another.

In total, we removed four full socks, along with the spoon—that's two full pairs of socks!

The owners had no idea any socks were missing, so I suppose it was lucky we performed the endoscopy and got a close look inside the dog's stomach, uncovering these additional objects along the way.

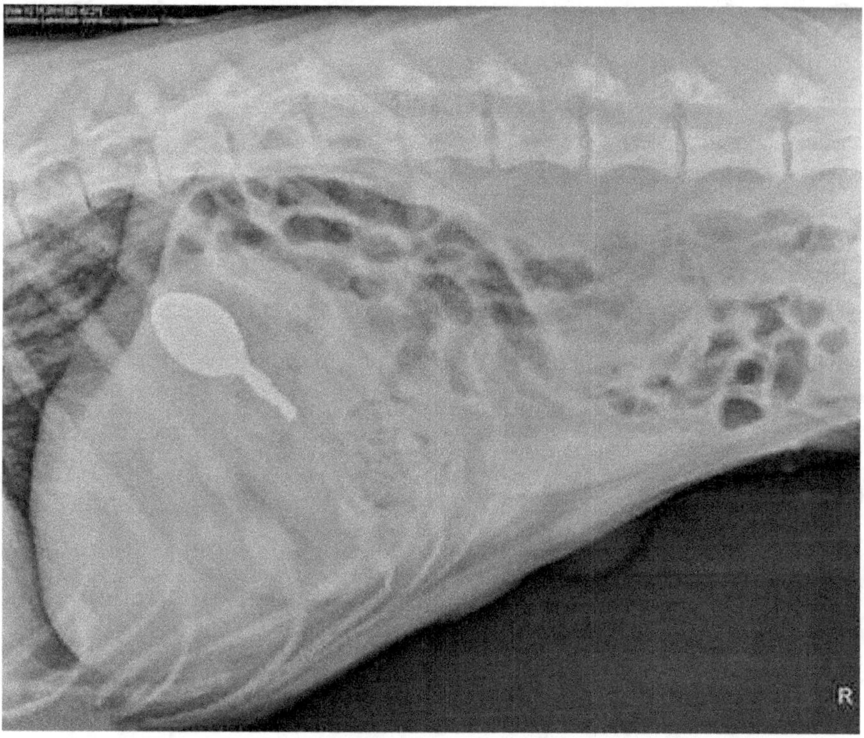

Figure 5. Peanut Butter on a Spoon

Chapter 5

Squishy the troublesome cat (Or, A Tale of Some Ties)

The list of "non-food items" that dogs and cats eat is long, endless, and often disgusting. Sometimes it's interesting or funny, but other times, it's just gross. In the ER, we regularly see the sick, the injured, and the dying… and that's what makes this job so difficult. We don't enjoy seeing animals become so ill, but we always do our best to help. Because the job can be so emotionally demanding, we learn to take joy in the small successes. Foreign bodies are one of those small victories that bring us a surprising amount of joy. They can represent a simple medical problem—often a potentially life-threatening one if left untreated—but the solution is usually straightforward, and the outcome is often amazing.

Gastrointestinal foreign bodies typically enter an animal in one way and exit in one of four: induced vomiting, endoscopy, surgery, or, in some lucky cases, they pass on their own. Some foreign bodies are easier to remove than others, depending on their size, shape, material, and where they're located in the body. When the object is still in the stomach, we can usually induce vomiting in dogs with a very high success rate over. Cats, however, are a different story. Despite their reputation for vomiting at home—hairballs, grass, or just to mess up your rug—getting a cat to vomit on cue with medication is far less successful. We have three different medications we can use in cats—dexmedetomidine, hydromorphone, and the less commonly used xylazine—all of which cause sedation and are reversible. But even with these tools, our success rate sits at only about 50%. That's right—just 50%! In veterinary medicine, this isn't unexpected. It's just one of the many ways different species respond differently. It's frustrating, and we often joke that cats follow their own rulebook. They rarely cooperate the way textbooks say they should, which makes treating them more difficult—but every now and then, they surprise us in the best ways. What follows is one of those good surprises, a moment where we got to celebrate a small but memorable victory.

Squishy, a five-year-old female cat, came in one evening brought by her young adult owners—vomiting, of course, as cats do. She was otherwise a healthy cat and had been seen by her primary vet just a week earlier for the same issue. At that visit, she had bloodwork done as part of her exam, and everything came back normal. The owners were unaware of anything she could have gotten into.

As always, we performed a thorough physical exam. Everything appeared fairly normal, with just two exceptions. She was a little dehydrated—likely from all the vomiting—and her belly felt a bit full. Not painful, just full, like she had eaten a large meal. She had arrived around 3 p.m., so as part of our history-taking, we asked, "When does she normally eat?" The owners told us she'd eaten about half of her usual meal that morning. We thought, "Maybe what we're feeling is just food in her stomach, but it does seem more distended than it should be." Since we weren't finding much on our physical exam, we continued asking questions. While it's far more common for dogs to eat non-food items, cats occasionally do can certainly do this as well.

So we asked, "Has she ever eaten any non-food items—medications, recreational or prescription drugs, toys, strings, anything like that?" The owners replied, "Nope, nothing."

We knew she needed supportive care. She wasn't sick enough to require hospitalization, so we discussed outpatient options. We planned to correct her dehydration with subcutaneous fluids and give her an antiemetic (anti-nausea medication) to help her feel better and, hopefully, stop the vomiting.

Still, the question remained: why was Squishy vomiting? Maybe something was in her stomach that didn't belong. So we recommended abdominal radiographs.

As always, we chose the next test with care—not just to run a test, but to gather meaningful information. After some discussion, the young couple agreed. They didn't have much money, so we had to be deliberate and thoughtful with every step, as costs can add up quickly (as we do every single day).

The nice thing about x-rays is that they're relatively simple. Most of the time, we take two views—called orthogonal views (sometimes we do three views). The first is taken with the patient lying on their side (usually the right), and the second with the patient on their back. The goal of taking these two perspectives is to visualize the internal organs more effectively. Since radiographs turn a three-dimensional animal into a two-dimensional image, we risk missing things if we only take one view.

Squishy's radiographs were interesting, to say the least (see Figures 6 and 7). Most of the abdominal contents looked normal, but the stomach appeared odd, which you can see in the image. Normally, when there's gas in the stomach—as there was here—we can see the rugal folds, which look like a series of squiggly lines. These folds exist because the stomach is a distensible organ. Like a balloon, it stretches when full, but when it's empty, it collapses into these accordion-like folds. When examining the radiographs, it looked like Squishy had an excessive number of rugal folds in her stomach—an uncommon finding. Another possibility was a large mass of worms. Either way, it was strange. Since Squishy had vomited recently, her stomach should have been relatively empty—unless, of course, something was in there that didn't belong.

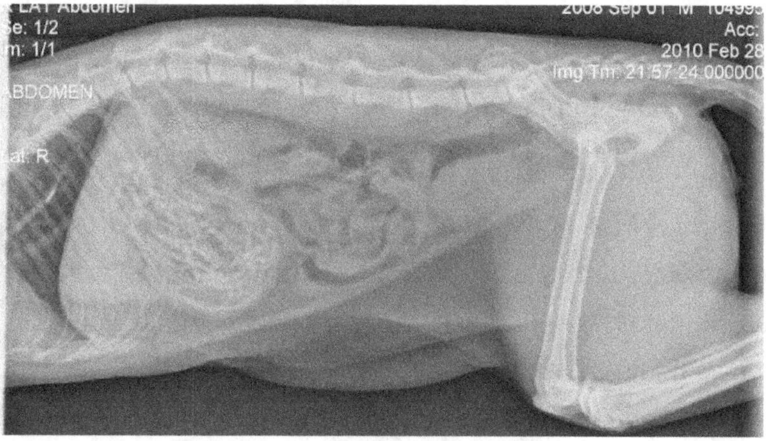

Figure 6.

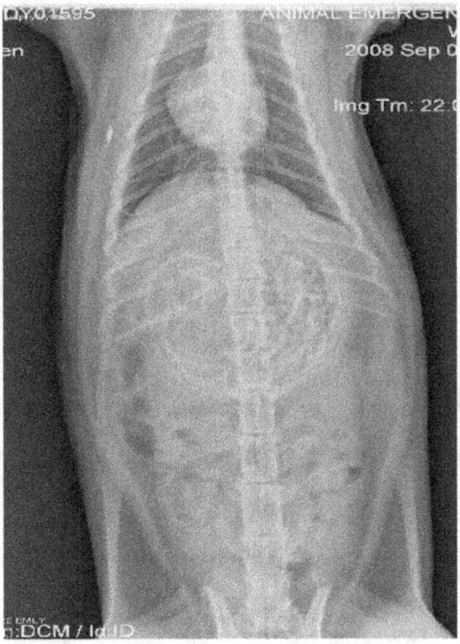

Figure 7.

As we reviewed the x-ray findings with the owners, we recommended further investigation into these “worm-like” structures visible in her stomach. The two options were endoscopy or surgery.

Surgery is a fairly straightforward choice—it gives us a definitive answer and allows us to take immediate action. If we didn’t find something obvious during surgery, we could still take biopsies of the stomach and intestines to investigate further. Endoscopy, while less invasive and a bit more affordable, doesn’t always yield a definitive diagnosis.

The young couple hesitated for a while as they considered their options. Ultimately, both of them called their parents—not just for advice, but also for financial support to help with Squishy’s unexpected medical crisis.

They decided to proceed with the endoscopy. I'll admit, I was a little hesitant myself. I wasn't fully confident that we'd get the answer we needed, but I was certainly willing to try.

Like every tool we use in medicine, no test or procedure is 100% guaranteed. Endoscopy is one of those tools—it has clear advantages, but also limitations. The endoscope is essentially a camera attached to the end of a flexible tube. We can maneuver the tip of the scope in all directions and pass small grasping tools through it, but using the endoscope effectively is a challenge, and takes some additional training. It's a bit like playing a video game—or like one of those arcade claw machines. Grabbing objects with the scope can vary substantially in the level of difficulty range from incredibly easy to nearly impossible. Imagine trying to thread a needle using tweezers controlled by a drone. It's doable—but not simple. That's what endoscopy is like.

We moved forward with the procedure. As with all veterinary patients, endoscopy requires general anesthesia. We placed an IV catheter and administered both injectable and inhaled anesthetics, along with oxygen. I always feel grateful to work in a hospital with access to advanced equipment—anesthetic monitors and endoscopy tools are just some of the "toys" that help us do our jobs well. These tools help ensure that our patients are safe and closely monitored during anesthesia.

Once Squishy was under anesthesia, we inserted the endoscope into her mouth, down her esophagus, and into her stomach. Instantly, the answer was clear. Her stomach appeared to be full of large black worms, all tangled together and slowly shifting with her breathing.

Now, cats don't really get worms in the stomach—at least not worms of that size—but that's exactly what it looked like. Upon closer inspection, though, we noticed that the "worms" weren't actually moving on their own. They were just swaying slightly with each breath.

We grasped one with the our endoscopy instrument and tried to pull it out. But it wouldn't come—whatever it was, it was entangled with the others. It stretched but wouldn't budge. We tried another, and then another—same result. Nothing would come out.

At that point, we called the owners again and brought up surgery. We could see the problem, but couldn't solve it with the scope. The owners, however, said they couldn't afford surgery and really hoped endoscopy would be enough. They still had faith in us and encouraged us to keep trying.

So we did.

We spent another twenty minutes grasping and pulling, trying different angles and approaches. Finally—success! We freed the first "worm". Once that one came out, we were able to maneuver it up the esophagus and out through the mouth. Then another followed… and another.

As we examined the first object, we realized it wasn't a worm at all—it was a hair tie. And so was the next one. And the next.

It turned out that Squishy had swallowed hair ties one by one, and they had become knotted and twisted together in her stomach, forming a tangled, stretchy mass. That's why they were so difficult to remove. The entire procedure ended up taking over two hours of anesthesia time.

In total, we removed **sixty-two hair ties** from Squishy's stomach. (See Figure 8.) Even now, I still can't quite believe it. Sixty-two. It was a long, probably uncomfortable procedure for Squishy, but we were thrilled to have solved the problem and avoided surgery. After confirming that there were no more hair ties left with some post-procedure x-rays, we recovered her from anesthesia and monitored her for several hours before sending her home. She drooled for about two days afterward, but eventually, she returned to normal and began eating again.

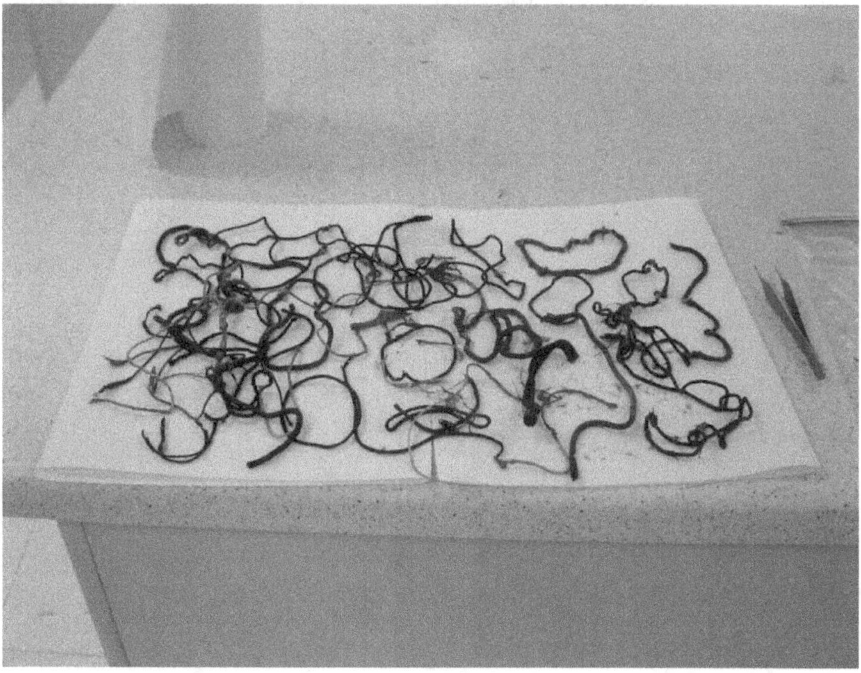

Figure 8.

Right after the procedure, we called the owners with the good news. They were both thrilled—and shocked.

The boyfriend laughed and said, "I thought she just kept losing them… I even bought her more because she was always running out!" Turns out, their cat had been silently hoarding them in her stomach, one at a time, until they finally caused a blockage.

For those who may not know, cats **love** to play with string-like objects—and they often swallow them. Thread, yarn, shoelaces, ribbon, rope, even hair ties—if a cat is willing to play with it, there's a good chance it might go down the hatch.

Needless to say, the owners tried to be much more careful after that

Chapter 6

Five bucks is a lot of cash to a kid!

So many things get ingested by dogs—it can be quite surprising. At the veterinary hospital, we regularly see patients who've eaten things they shouldn't. Often, it's food that's inappropriate for dogs. Sometimes it's harmless, like lunch meat or bread, but many everyday household items can be dangerous or even toxic. Chocolate and onions are well-known examples, but there are lesser-known culprits too, like bread dough, sugar-free gum, and grapes or raisins.

Dogs are curious creatures. Like infants, they have limited ways to explore the world, which often means putting things in their mouths—and sometimes swallowing them before anyone has a chance to react.

As I've mentioned before, when animals eat something they shouldn't, we only have a few options to remove the object (let it pass, induce vomiting, endoscopy [which we just reviewed in the previous story], or surgery). If it's small and not dangerous, we can sometimes wait for it to pass. That's what I had to do once when I was younger.

When I was about twelve years old, I had a paper route (like, very cliche, but a job that existed in the past). For several years, I got up at 5 a.m., gathered the newspapers, slung my burlap bag over my shoulder, and delivered them house to house. At the end of each month, I'd go back door to door to collect payment. Back then, most people paid in cash. I'd pay the newspaper company what I owed, and the rest was mine to keep as profit.

So, every month, I had a small stack of cash that I carefully organized, counted, and stored—at least, I thought I stored it safely. As a twelve-year-old, I didn't really consider that my dog might eat money. One day, while recounting my stash, I noticed that one of my $10 bills was torn in half, with ragged edges.

Now, when you're a kid, $10 is a lot of money (or ast least it was back then), and I wanted to know what happened to it. I showed my parents, and they immediately suspected the dog. We found her—Jasper, the same dog I mentioned earlier—lying innocently in the hallway. We opened her mouth and, sure enough, found a tiny piece of paper wedged between her teeth. Jasper was my best friend growing up, and I couldn't believe she'd betray me like that!

Well, what was done was done, and the money was gone—or so we thought.

That $10 was important to me, and I wanted to recover as much as I could. So off to the bank we went. If you've ever tried to exchange a torn bill at the bank, you know they won't replace the full amount unless you have most of the bill. They measure how much of it you have, give you that portion in cash, and send the rest to the Treasury for destruction.

I brought my half of the $10 bill that remained to the bank in a little plastic bag and explained the situation to the teller. I told her my dog had eaten the other half and we were sure it was destroyed. I asked if I could get the full $10.

They said, “No, we’ll give you $5, since you’ve got about half of it.” I understand it now, but at the time, that $5 was a big deal—it was part of my hard-earned profits. I said, “Okay,” and walked home, head hanging low, with my five dollars. I’m sure my parents thought it was a valuable lesson in responsibility.

But I wasn’t done yet!

Being a responsible dog owner, I was in charge of picking up the poop in our backyard every week. I figured, if Jasper really swallowed the rest of that bill, maybe—just maybe—it could still come out the other end. I asked my mom, who was a nurse at the time, and she explained that paper might be able to pass through the intestines, but warned me not to get my hopes up. She said Jasper might have chewed it up too much, or it could be digested—or lost entirely.

But of course, I got my hopes up. Surely half of a $10 bill could survive a trip through the GI tract of a dog, right? That week, I dutifully checked Jasper’s poop every day. Four days later, I noticed one pile looked… different. Something was crumpled inside.

I grabbed some rubber gloves and the garden hose and picked that poop apart. And believe it or not—I found it! The other half of the $10 bill had made it through her stomach and colon, and was still intact!

I carefully cleaned it off, flattened it out, and placed it in another little plastic bag. I ran into the house yelling, “I found it! I found it!” I explained what had happened to my parents, and the next day after school, we went back to the bank.

I really wish I had photos from that day, but unfortunately, I don't. I am quite sure, however, that the bank teller had never heard a story like mine. I explained that the first half of the bill had been rejected, so I went on a mission to find the second half. Her expression was priceless as I handed over that poop-salvaged half of a $10 bill in its plastic bag.

I'm sure she had a story to tell her coworkers: about how a ten-dollar bill made its way through the digestive tract of a dog and ended up back at the bank. Hey, at least I cleaned it off first! And the look on my face was probably just as memorable as I walked out of the bank—proudly holding my other five dollars.

Chapter 7

That underwear is not mine!

Now we move on to explore one of the other ways to remove foreign objects: surgery. Obviously, we only take this route when other options have failed, or when it's the only viable choice. For example, if something is lodged in the middle of the intestines, it can't be removed by inducing emesis, nor can it be reached with an endoscope—the intestines are simply too long and narrow. In these cases, we have to perform surgery to retrieve the object.

This story begins with Finnely, a four-year-old Golden Retriever who came into the clinic—bouncy as ever and not feeling too bad. His owners reported that he had been vomiting for two days and hadn't eaten much. I performed a physical examination and noted some mild abdominal pain. After a short discussion, I recommended we take radiographs of his abdomen to see if we could identify the cause of his vomiting. Sometimes radiographs are helpful, and sometimes they're not. This time, we got lucky.

The radiographs showed something suspicious in the middle of his intestines—causing significant dilation and likely an obstruction. We could also faintly see something with a streaky, gas-trapping pattern, which suggested the presence of fabric. This is not always visible on radiographs—textile materials like socks or washcloths often don't show up clearly—but in Finnely's case, the signs pointed strongly to something stuck in there.

I reviewed the findings with the owner and went over our options. I always emphasize that when there's concern for an intestinal obstruction, the recommendation is surgery. If the intestines become blocked, blood supply can be compromised and the tissue begins to die. This is called necrosis, and it can lead to intestinal contents leaking into the abdominal cavity—resulting in a life-threatening infection known as septic peritonitis. Without hesitation, the owner agreed that we should proceed to surgery immediately.

It takes some time to prepare a dog for surgery. We have to place an intravenous catheter to administer anesthetic drugs and fluids. We also run pre-anesthetic bloodwork to ensure it's safe to proceed. Fortunately, aside from some mild dehydration, Finnely's bloodwork came back normal. We started IV fluids while prepping the surgical suite.

I work in a multi-doctor practice with several veterinary assistants and technicians. Anytime there's news of an interesting surgery—especially a foreign body removal—word spreads quickly. Everyone either pops into the OR or peers through the window to see what strange item the dog may have swallowed. Finnely's case was no exception. Those who've worked with me long enough know that when they ask, "What is it?" my usual reply is simply, "A foreign body." I'm not sure if I say that to keep the suspense going, to avoid distractions, or simply because my focus is on the patient, the surgery, and the anesthesia.

Sometimes, even I don't know what the foreign object is until it's out. Most fabric-based foreign bodies are wadded up, discolored, and coated in intestinal contents—making identification difficult at first glance. We also minimize handling the object during surgery, using sterile instruments and gloves, since it's contaminated with intestinal bacteria. We always complete the procedure first before doing a closer inspection. If it's fabric, it might turn out to be a sock, underwear, part of a towel, a carpet scrap—who knows?

We were very fortunate with Finnely. His owners brought him in quickly and consented to surgery without delay. We were able to remove the obstruction with a single incision into the intestine. There was no evidence of rupture, and he tolerated anesthesia well. His recovery was smooth—he was comfortable on pain medication and began eating on his own just hours after the surgery. He met all the post-op milestones we hope for, and we were able to send him home shortly thereafter. We were thrilled with how smoothly it all went!

As I mentioned earlier, most foreign bodies we remove are fairly disgusting—coated in intestinal juices, blood, and smelling awful. They're often compacted into tight, unrecognizable clumps. Finnely's was no different.

Of course, just like the staff, the owners usually want to know what the foreign object was. After surgery, I donned gloves, washed off the object, and unfolded it. What I found was... a piece of lady's underwear. Skimpy, frilly, and lacy. More specifically: a red lace thong.

The next morning, during visiting hours before Finnely's discharge, both of his owners—husband and wife—came to see him. Naturally, they asked to see the foreign body.I pulled out the underwear—carefully contained in a plastic baggie—and showed it to the couple. The female owner immediately turned the same color as the underwear. Red in the face and clearly embarrassed, she looked away. I tried to ease the tension, explaining that this wasn't uncommon. As I've said before, dogs can be gross. Eating underwear—especially dirty underwear—is, unfortunately, not unusual. They sniff it, lick it, pull it from the hamper or off the floor, and before you know it, it's been swallowed!

At first, she seemed to relax a little and took a closer look at the underwear. Then, suddenly, her face turned a different shade of red—an angrier one, like a spark had been lit in her eyes. She turned to her husband and said, with ice in her voice, "Dear, this underwear is NOT MINE."

At that point, I quickly excused myself and my staff from the room before things got ugly. I gently escorted the owners out of the ICU and into an exam room with Finnely so they could continue their visit—and their conversation—in private.

Of course, many staff members in the clinic had overheard her declaration, and speculation began flying. "Was there another woman in the picture?" "Did the mom forget she owned this pair?" Our minds were racing.

We'll never know exactly what was said between them, but we certainly heard some yelling at first. It sounded like a heated argument, and while I couldn't say who was winning, she definitely had some choice words for him. After a few minutes, things went quiet.

What I hadn't mentioned yet was that the owners had planned for the rest of their family to visit that day as well. Their two children—

a 12-year-old boy and a 17-year-old girl—arrived later that afternoon to see Finnely after his surgery. And naturally, they had the same question: "What was removed?"

Mom shot a sharp look at Dad. He looked down—maybe ashamed, maybe just stunned. Then, clearly uncomfortable, Mom reached into her bag and pulled out the little plastic pouch to show her kids the recovered item.

A blood-curdling scream erupted from the room. "Oh my God!!"

I immediately ran in, worried that something had gone wrong with Finnely—was he in pain? Had his sutures opened up? But just as I opened the door, the daughter bolted past me, tears in her eyes—and, just like her mother earlier, she was as red as the underwear.

Despite all our early speculation—whether Dad was cheating or hiding something—we soon discovered the truth: the little, lacy red underwear belonged to their daughter.

It was a bit awkward, but thankfully, no real harm was done. The family got past the embarrassment, and Finnely? He lived to eat another day… hopefully with no more red thongs on the menu!

Chapter 8

Milking things…. it's not just for cows anymore

Where does this story begin? Probably not where you'd expect. I started it with a title about milking cows, so let's start there.

Modern dairy farms are impressive. They treat their cows well, produce a lot of milk, and manage their place in the food chain responsibly. Milking machines must be pristinely maintained—sterile, safe, efficient, and comfortable for the cow. It's quite a sight to see a large, well-run dairy operation and how resourceful and productive it can be. Milking cows is a major industry in the U.S., and most of us benefit from it daily. Here, we also milk other species. Goats, for instance, have their own modest milk industry. A few other species are milked too—but the rest of this story is about "milking" something very different.

I'm not talking about collecting milk from cows or goats with a machine. I'm talking about the physical act of manually pushing something out of a tube-like structure by hand. In the small animal hospital, that's what we mean when we talk about "milking."

But let's back up a bit—to where the verb actually comes from. As a veterinary student, I spent time on farms and learned how to milk a cow by hand. In vet school, we take a class that includes animal husbandry and production medicine. There, we learn how cows are prepped for milking machines, how to collect milk samples to test for disease, hormones, or antibiotic residues, and how to assess the animals' overall health. It's important to learn how to milk properly—to get the sample without causing harm to the cow or goat. There's a technique: a firm but gentle pinch and squeeze. Too hard, and the cow finds it unpleasant; too soft, and you don't get the prize—whole milk.

Large animal vets do this regularly to collect samples, but I don't do it much these days. Still, you never know when a skill like that might come in handy. Because "milking" isn't just for teats (yes, that's the correct medical term)—it's a technique that works for a variety of organs.

As I mentioned, in the small animal hospital, "milking" usually refers to pushing something along or out of a hollow organ—like the intestines, bladder, or gallbladder. Usually, we're trying to extract something that doesn't belong there. The most common things we milk out are either foreign objects from the intestines or stones from the urinary tract.

When an animal has a foreign object in its intestines and needs surgery, it's common for us to have to "milk" that object up or down the tract for various reasons. I've done this so many times with dogs and cats that it's hard to know where to begin—but let's go with the story of a dog named Lucy.

Lucy was a young golden-doodle mix who came into our emergency room every month for five months in a row. Like clockwork. Five months. She had a very specific habit—and a very specific taste: lady's underwear. Need I say more about the timing of her visits? Probably not for the female readers. For the men reading,

I'll clarify: Lucy's visits coincided with one of the female household members' menstrual cycle.

Poor Lucy. I'm not sure who in the house was responsible for leaving the laundry basket accessible—maybe the husband, the wife, or one of the kids—but someone kept giving Lucy access. You'd think they'd learn after the first time. Or maybe the second. But no—it took five emergency visits before they fully accepted that Lucy could not be trusted with laundry.

Over the course of those five months, we used a variety of techniques to get the underwear out. Twice, it was easy—the owners brought her in quickly, and we induced vomiting. Out came light blue and green skimpy underwear. Twice, vomiting didn't work, so we had to perform endoscopy—those times, she'd swallowed red and black pairs. Apparently, Lucy had favorites.

The fifth, and most expensive, visit required surgery. The underwear was lodged way down in the intestines, and we had to open her abdominal cavity. We made an incision in the intestines and removed the final pair—pink, this time. That's where our "milking" technique came in; we had to carefully move the underwear through the intestines toward the surgical incision in the healthiest segment.

Let me explain why we sometimes need to milk foreign bodies during surgery. Occasionally, we can milk the object backward from the intestines into the stomach; when we can make an incision into the stomach instead of the intestines, it's better for the patient. Stomach incisions come with fewer potential complications—it's a forgiving organ, distensible, with extra tissue, and we can close it in two layers. The intestines, on the other hand, are more delicate and only get a single-layer closure.

In some cases, we try to milk the object forward through the ileocecal junction—the valve connecting the small intestines to the colon. Foreign objects often get stuck there. If we can successfully move the object into the colon, we may not need to make any incisions at all—once in the colon, it usually passes with the stool. Again, much better for the patient.

Sometimes, however, the object is lodged squarely in the middle of the intestines, and in those cases, we have no choice but to make an incision close to where the foreign material is stuck. When we make an incision into the intestine, we do so on the side of the intestinal "tube" opposite the blood vessels, to maintain healthy blood flow and optimize healing. A foreign body stuck in the intestines can cause severe bruising, inflammation, and even compromise the blood supply, so we always try to make the incision in the healthiest-looking portion of the intestines—often just beyond or just before the object. The healthier the tissue, the lower the risk of complications.

There are also times we encounter foreign bodies, particularly linear ones (like string or fabric), that span a large portion of the gastrointestinal tract—from stomach to colon. In those situations, we often have to make multiple incisions; we do our best to make as few and as short of incisions as possible to minimize surgical time and risk.

Even when surgery is done properly, there's always a small risk that the incision may not heal correctly, a complication known as dehiscence. After closing intestinal incisions with suture, we even perform a “leak test” by injecting sterile saline into the lumen of the intestine to ensure no contents leak out, but ultimately, we’re relying on the patient’s own ability to heal. When an incision fails to heal, the intestinal contents can spill into the abdominal cavity, leading to a potentially life-threatening condition called sepsis. It’s a rare event—but when it occurs, it can become a disaster if not caught early.

So why bring all this up? Because every time we cut into the intestines, we carry these risks in mind. Several published studies have examined the factors that increase the likelihood of dehiscence. These include the part of the GI tract involved (the colon has the highest risk, followed by the small intestine, then the stomach), underlying intestinal disease (like inflammatory bowel disease or damage caused by the foreign body itself), and intraoperative complications such as low blood pressure—which is one reason we monitor patients so closely under anesthesia.

Back to Lucy’s surgery. As mentioned, a foreign object that causes a complete intestinal obstruction can block the blood supply and distend the intestines. So, when we had to make an incision to retrieve the underwear she’d swallowed, we chose the healthiest portion of the intestine and used our milking skills to guide the object toward the opening. That final pair—pink—was gently coaxed through her intestines until we could remove it cleanly from our single incision site.

There’s a certain finesse required when milking something through the intestines. You can only apply so much pressure before risking further damage. It’s not a skill you can measure precisely—

it's more art than science. It can't be taught from a textbook; it's something you learn from experience and feel.

And sometimes, those milking skills come in handy with more unusual species.

One day, I had to use them in the most unexpected way. In fact, I've got two stories—both involving animals we rarely see in a small animal hospital—where milking made all the difference.

The first begins with a cria. If you're unfamiliar with the term, a *cria* is a baby alpaca. And yes, you might be wondering what a small animal veterinarian like me was doing treating an alpaca. The answer is: we rarely do. In fact, this is probably the only alpaca I've treated since becoming a licensed vet.

It was a late evening, when most veterinary hospitals—especially large animal facilities—were closed. That's when we often receive calls for cases that have nowhere else to go. I've always said I'll treat any patient as long as we can safely restrain it (for example, I can't hold down a cow or a tiger nor restrain them properly in my small animla hospital) and the animal doesn't pose an undue risk to our staff (no venomous snakes... or tigers, obviously).

The owner on the phone explained that they had been syringe-feeding their young cria, who was struggling to nurse and failing to gain weight. They'd been using a red rubber feeding tube—about 18 inches long—inserted through her mouth and into the esophagus. But during one feeding, the tube slipped off the end of the syringe and slid down her throat. The cria was repeatedly swallowing, likely trying to move the tube deeper into her esophagus or into her stomach.

When they brought her in, she was young, a bit underweight, but otherwise her physical exam was normal. She was swallowing a lot, which was concerning—but also, oddly helpful. The challenge: I'd never treated an alpaca before, let alone a juvenile one. And alpacas have *long* necks—hers was close to two feet. How would I retrieve a feeding tube from *that*?

Luckily, one of our staff veterinarians had experience in large animal medicine and was just finishing her shift. She offered guidance on which sedatives we could use safely (since not all medications translate across species). We were hoping to avoid endoscopy, as the cost was a concern for the owner. Our hope was that the tube might still be visible in the back of the mouth, so we could retrieve it without invasive equipment.

We sedated the cria with intramuscular injections, and the medication worked well. Though I couldn't see the tube at the back of her mouth, her relaxed neck muscles allowed me to palpate deeply—and I could actually *feel* the tube inside her esophagus! So, I put those trusty milking skills to work.

Gently, inch by inch, I began to milk the rubber tube up her neck. Eventually, it reached high enough in her throat that we could just see the tip peeking out in the back of her mouth. Using a long surgical instrument, I grasped it and pulled it free!

We had the tube out, the cria feeling better, and the whole visit took under an hour. She even let out a little bleat on her way out the door—cute as can be, symptom-free, and headed home.The final story I have about these exceptional milking skills involves yet another unusual species—and, yes, it's a snake.

Now, have you ever heard the term *milking a snake*? Traditionally, that refers to extracting venom from a venomous snake—something performed by highly trained professionals. I've never treated a venomous snake (and honestly, I don't ever plan to). They're illegal to own in most parts of the country, and for good reason. You'd think we wouldn't need laws to tell people not to keep venomous snakes in their homes... but, well, the world is full of very *interesting* individuals.

When venom is collected from snakes, it's typically used to develop antivenins that help treat animals and people who've been bitten. Dogs, horses, cats, and humans are all occasional victims of snake bites, and antivenins can be life-saving. Thankfully, we don't see many snakebite cases where I practice in Wisconsin, but now I've moved to Colorado, we see snake bites all the time—again, maybe I'll share more on that another time.

This particular story, however, doesn't involve venom collection. But it does involve a snake. And it *does* involve milking—just not in the traditional sense.

The call came from our local urban ecology center about a four-and-a-half-foot bullsnake—non-venomous, thank goodness. The center keeps a few local wildlife species to help educate the public about which animals are native, which are dangerous, and how to tell them apart.

On this particular day, the center's volunteers—two responsible teenagers—were feeding the snake her usual diet of thawed frozen mice. Following proper safety protocols, they wore thick leather gloves while offering the mouse—just in case she decided to nip at the hand that feeds her. While bullsnakes aren't venomous, a bite can still hurt and lead to infection.

But on this day, the snake was especially eager—and instead of just grabbing the mouse, she grabbed the entire *gloved hand.* She bit down, yanked the glove off, and began coiling around it. Then she started swallowing it.

"Why would she do that?" you might ask. Well, consider that the glove had just been holding a dead mouse and probably smelled strongly of her usual food. She likely thought she was being served an extra-large meal. This behavior was not abnormal for a snake—just inconvenient.

The teens tried to help. They gently attempted to pull the glove out of her mouth. But every time they did, she clamped down harder and swallowed faster. Realizing that they were only making the situation worse, they did the right thing: they stopped, and they called us.

We asked them to bring her in immediately—before she swallowed the entire glove.

They placed her carefully into a hard-sided cooler and rushed her over. But despite their best efforts to get to us quickly, by the time they arrived, it was too late. We opened the cooler—and no glove was in sight.

Now, usually, after a snake eats a meal, you can spot a distinct bulge in the body where the food is being digested. But this snake was a heavy-bodied girl, and no matter how we looked or palpated, we couldn't find a bulge large enough to suggest an entire adult-sized leather glove was inside her.

So our first step was to make sure we weren't chasing a red herring—or glove. We asked again: "Are you absolutely certain she was swallowing the glove when you placed her in the cooler?"

And they confirmed it. Absolutely. They saw it in her mouth.Well, we couldn't feel it, but we were confident it was in there somewhere.

A quick anatomy lesson on snakes: if you sliced one into cross-sections (like a cucumber), they're roughly shaped like the letter "C." Their vertebrae and back muscles form the closed portion of the C, while their soft abdominal contents make up the open side—of course, all wrapped in scales. When their muscles contract, their bodies feel firm and solid. But when they relax, you can actually slip your fingers into that open "C" shape to feel around inside. Even with a deep palpation, though, we couldn't feel the glove. And to make matters worse, the snake was getting very enthusiastic about all this attention—squirming, flexing, and making the job increasingly difficult.

Since palpation didn't help, we turned to an x-ray. To do that, we needed to sedate her. At the time, we had recently acquired a new injectable anesthetic agent called alfaxalone, which was safe for use in reptiles. We drew up a dose and injected it into her muscles. Over the next 10 to 15 minutes, she started to relax and become drowsy. With another deep palpation, we *thought* we could feel something unusual that might be the glove, but we weren't sure—so we proceeded with radiographs.

In the image (Figure 9), the snake is curled around the outer edge of the x-ray plate. We believed we could make out the faint outline of the glove. That gave us the confirmation we needed—it was in there.

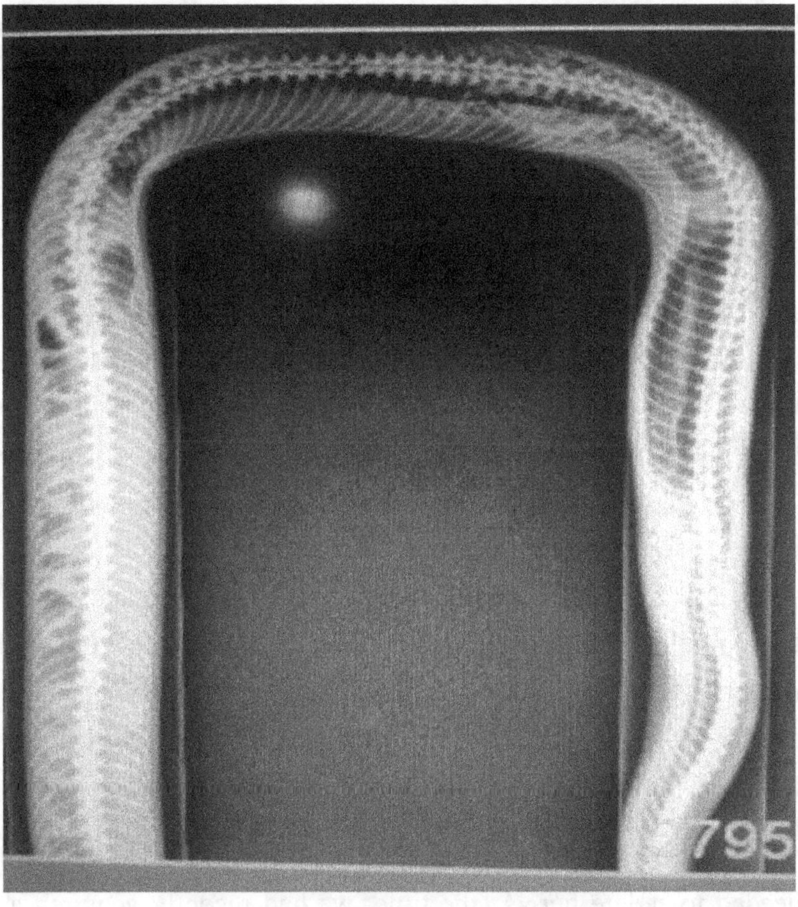

Figure 9.

Now the real question was:

How were we going to get it out?

Milking!

Once again, those milking techniques were about to come in handy.

Since she was nice and sedate, we decided to try milking the glove *backwards* out of her. This method shouldn't harm her—after all, snakes sometimes regurgitate meals naturally. So, like squeezing a large, scale-covered tube of toothpaste, we got to work gently working the glove back up her body, toward her mouth.

At first, she tolerated the process well. We made steady progress, slowly moving the glove toward her throat. But once it reached her glottis (the opening at the back of the throat), she was *not* happy. Her sedation started wearing off, and she began writhing and resisting.

We had mistakenly thought this would be a straightforward process—it wasn't.

We kept squeezing, carefully but persistently, and started making progress again. But then the "tube of toothpaste" fought back. She began using her powerful muscles to try and swallow the glove back down. She was determined to keep it. Now, we were working against her and against the natural flow of digestion. It felt like pushing a rock uphill.

Eventually, we managed to push the glove far enough forward that we could *see* the tip at the back of her throat. But just as quickly, she started swallowing again—and the glove began disappearing from view.

Worried about getting our fingers bitten, we needed a tool—fast.

“Someone bring us a hemostat!” I shouted. “Oh my goodness—it’s right there!” I could see the glove slipping back down, just past her glottis. We were losing it.

In the nick of time, one of my assistants handed me the hemostat. I reached in, grabbed the glove, and slowly pulled it from her mouth. **Success!**

Cheers erupted in the ER.

There’s something universally satisfying about pulling a foreign object out of a patient. The room filled with sighs of relief. I’m pretty sure I was sweating, but I was so grateful we didn’t have to resort to scoping or surgery.

The snake herself gave what looked like a big sigh—yes, you could actually *see* her breathe out. Then, she slept off the rest of her anesthesia for the next four hours while we all laughed about the absurdity of the situation.

Below, you’ll see some pictures showing the size of the snake and the adult leather glove we managed to retrieve from her. Figure 10 shows the glove as it emerged, and Figure 11 shows it fully unwrapped.

The snake returned to her important job the very next day, teaching visitors about local wildlife. And just to prove she was feeling fine, she ate another mouse—no hesitation.

The ecology center, having learned a valuable lesson, retired their leather gloves and started using large feeding tongs instead.

And as for us? Our milking skills were now certified.

Anyone for a glass of milk?

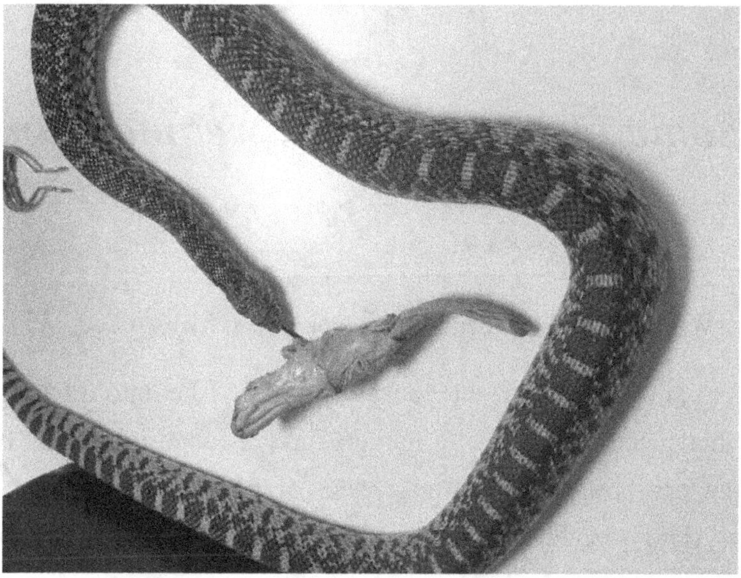

Figure 10

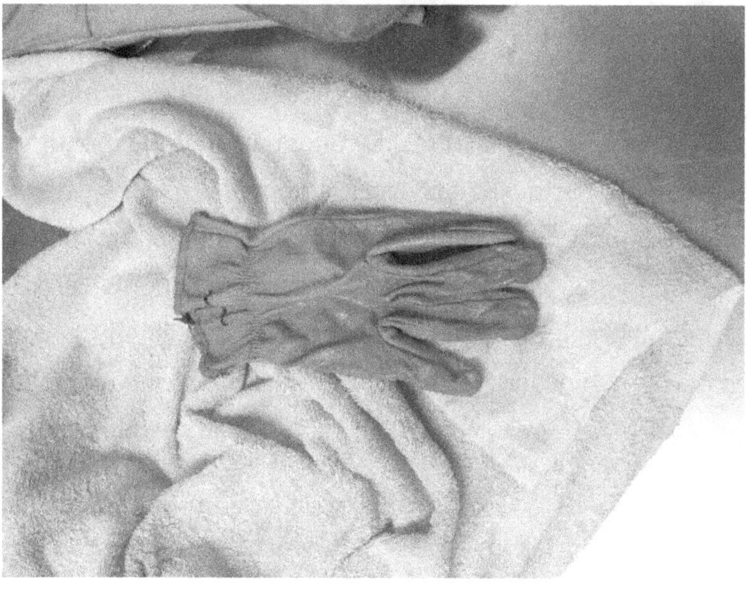

Figure 11

Chapter 9

Some feel good times: wet meat and a screw

Well, it was Memorial Day weekend in Milwaukee, Wisconsin.

A short review of the backstory before I get into the (wet) meat of this success story: veterinarians have a tough job, and I had just come off one of the worst weeks of my career—a week where everything seemed to come together in the worst possible way. I was feeling emotionally drained and, frankly, somewhat depressed. I'm a resilient person, so this kind of mood usually lasts only a couple of days, but it was hitting me hard. I didn't even want to go in to work.

Why was I feeling this way? Well, I had just finished a long stretch of days in a row and had worked most of the month without a single day off. Seriously—no exaggeration here. This is a big problem in the veterinary profession, and it's something many of us face at some point in our careers. There's currently a nationwide shortage of veterinarians, and the demand for services—especially in emergency medicine—has never been higher. Most veterinary hospitals have seen a 150% or greater increase in caseload over the past several years.

You might think veterinary staff work 9–5, but that's far from the truth—especially in an ER. In that long, exhausting month, I was completing medical records at home, coming in on my "days off" to catch up on work, and constantly putting out fires. I was exhausted.

But overwork wasn't the only reason I was feeling so low. As a specialist, I perform a lot of diagnostic ultrasound examinations. Ultrasound uses high-frequency sound waves to look inside the body, usually the abdomen. It's not necessarily "better" than radiographs—it simply gives different information. Ultrasound lets us look inside organs in a non-invasive way, and it's certainly less expensive than something like a CT scan.

In the previous seven days, I had performed about 25 ultrasounds. The diagnoses ranged from foreign bodies and gastroenteritis to cancer and kidney or liver disease. Some outcomes were hopeful. Most were not. Unfortunately, in that single week, 20 of those patients—80%—were diagnosed with cancer.

Now, cancer in dogs and cats isn't always a hopeless diagnosis. These days, there are many treatment options. Palliative care can provide comfort for a time, and aggressive treatments like chemotherapy, surgery, and even radiation can significantly improve both quality and length of life. Advances in veterinary oncology in recent years have been incredible. Contrary to popular belief, chemotherapy often causes few side effects in our patients, post-surgical pain is usually short-lived and well-managed, and radiation is non-invasive altogether.

But that week was different. All 20 cancer patients had already experienced metastasis—the cancer had spread to other organs. This meant the disease was likely aggressive and the prognosis poor.

Delivering that much bad news in such a short time was emotionally exhausting.

Adding to that burden, we had a two-year-old cat with a life-threatening infection pass away in the ICU. It's relatively uncommon for our patients to die from their illness, so when it happens, we take it hard. This cat's name was Tinsel. She had eaten a piece of string and undergone surgery at her primary care vet to remove it. Unfortunately, when string gets stuck in the intestines, it can act like a saw, cutting through the tissue. In Tinsel's case, the damage was severe, and the surgical incisions into her intestines broke down (a complication called dehiscence), leading to a devastating infection. We tried everything, but it wasn't enough.

So that was the somber backdrop heading into the holiday weekend. By Sunday night, after another 14+ hour shift and being on call all weekend for one of our busiest times of the year, I was finally wrapping things up to go home. But I wasn't exactly looking forward to it—my fiancée (now my wife) was away visiting her family out of state, so home meant being alone.

Just as I was winding down, one of our interns was examining a dog who had come in with some mild respiratory distress. This was a 7-month-old Golden Retriever named Charlie, and his case would change my mood entirely.

Charlie had been making "gurgling" and "snorting" noises for the past day. For such a young dog to come to the ER for breathing trouble was unusual. The way he was breathing suggested something stuck in the back of his nose. The owner's account shed more light—and added a much-needed dash of humor.

Charlie had been staying at a pet-sitter's house where all the dogs were given a "Pup-peroni" treat the day before his symptoms began. (If you don't know, Pup-peroni is like a Slim Jim for dogs.) Charlie swallowed his treat in one gulp—biting it only once—and promptly vomited. That's when the strange breathing started.

By the time he came to us, Charlie had already been to his primary care vet, who prescribed anti-inflammatories and antibiotics, but the symptoms persisted. He'd also visited another emergency clinic, where they determined the issue was in his nose and attempted a nasal flush. No luck. So he ended up at our hospital.

On exam, Charlie couldn't breathe with his mouth closed, had some mucoid discharge from one nostril, and was producing stertor (a snortling sound) when trying to breathe—all signs of a nasal or upper airway obstruction. His adorableness was undeniable; in the pictures we took (Figures 12 and 13), you can see him holding his own leash—of course, in Green Bay Packers colors.

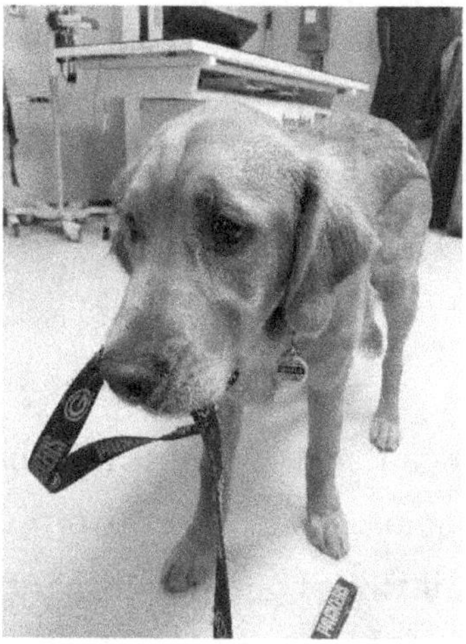

Figures 12

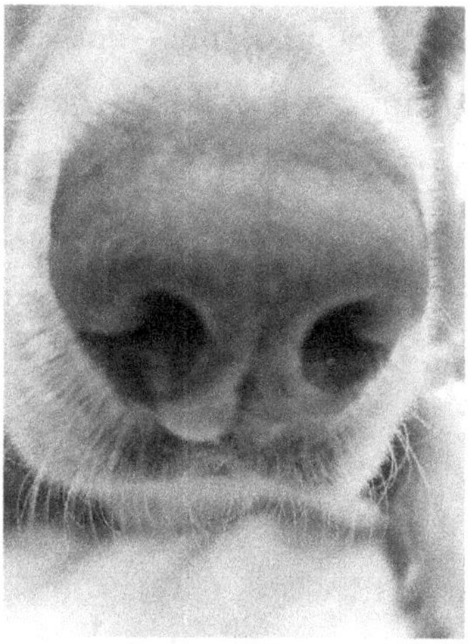

Figures 13

After hearing his history, we kept our theory simple: what if, when Charlie vomited, the Pup-peroni had somehow ended up in the back of his nasal cavity instead of coming out of his mouth? And what if it was still stuck there? Flushing hadn't worked, so we'd have to try something else.

A quick anatomy lesson: a dog's mouth is easy to access—you can open it, see inside, and feel around. But the nose is another matter entirely. It's a long tube with two tiny holes (the nostrils) in the front and a small opening in the back called the nasopharynx. This is separated from the mouth by the soft palate, and surrounded by bone and delicate structures called nasal turbinates—coiled loops of tissue that warm and humidify the air. In short, you can't easily see into a dog's nasal cavity, and you certainly can't reach in there with your fingers or standard instruments.

It was, in other words, a perplexing situation.

We're lucky at our hospital to have advanced medical tools for tricky cases like this—one of the most useful being endoscopy. Endoscopy is a flexible camera that lets us look behind the nose, and it can pass grasping instruments through it. This scope can actually turn 180 degrees to look back on itself or, in this case, peer above the soft palate into the nasopharynx. For Charlie, this was going to be the perfect tool.

However, there was a complication: the Pup-peroni had been soaking in mucus in the back of his nose for a day or two. Even with the largest endoscopy instruments, it wasn't going to be easy to grab. By now, the treat—what we started calling "wet meat"—had lost its structure. Instead of a cohesive piece of meat, it had become friable, crumbly… almost like ground beef.

The situation was like this: imagine using remote-control tweezers to pull a 2-inch glob of uncooked ground beef that's been sitting in milk through a straw, and then placing it into a cup in another room. Not fun. But that was exactly what we had to do.

The owners were eager for us to help Charlie. As usual, we placed an IV catheter, administered anesthesia, and intubated him. We inserted the flexible scope through his mouth, retroflexed it into the back of his nose, and there it was. A large, bloody glob of wet meat, blocking his airway from behind (See Figure 14).

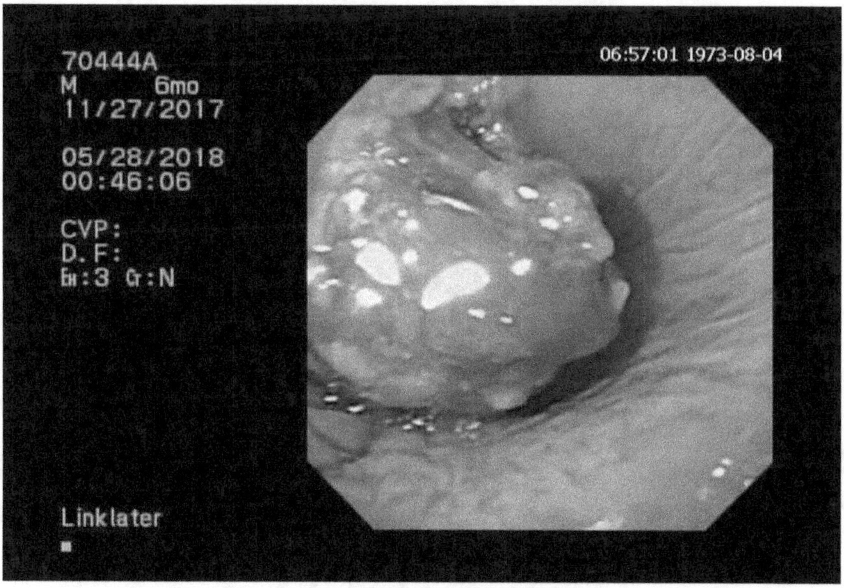

Figures 14

I tried grasping it, but just as expected, it crumbled. After twenty minutes of failed attempts, it was time to get creative. We passed a Foley catheter—a tube with a small balloon at the tip—through the nostril to the back of the nose, inflated it, and tried pushing from the front while pulling with the scope from behind. Our first "success" was pulling out a small piece… but when we looked again, the Pupperoni had split into two pieces.

After another twenty or thirty minutes of careful positioning, we finally got enough traction to move the larger piece from the back of the nose into the mouth. Once it reached the back of the throat, I could simply grab it with my hand and remove it. **SUCCESS!** The final haul: two pieces, about 1 cm wide and 5 cm long (see Figure 15).

It was deeply satisfying to have a win with a young dog after such a rough weekend. Even though it meant staying late, it was worth it. But before I could leave, the phone rang. Snowy was on her way.

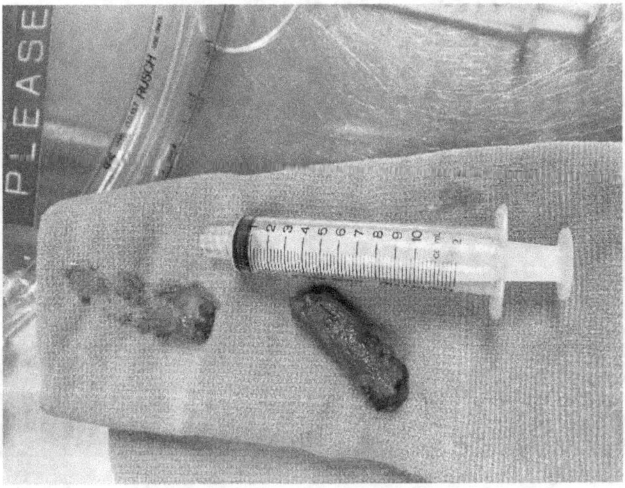

Figures 15

Snowy, another young Golden Retriever, and appropriately blonde (Figure 16), had swallowed a small, sharp-ended metal screw. At another emergency clinic, they tried to make her vomit—twice—but the screw stayed put. They decided it was too risky to wait for it to pass naturally and referred her to us for endoscopy. Since I was on call, this one was mine, too.

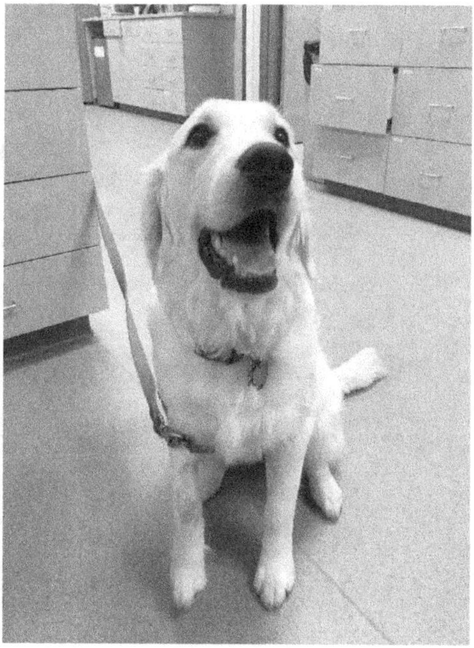

Figures 16

Removing a sharp metal object from a stomach without causing damage is delicate work. After reviewing the X-rays, we sedated Snowy and carefully maneuvered the endoscopy tools to grasp the screw. It took several tries, but eventually we pulled it into a protective tube so it wouldn't scratch or puncture anything on the way out. Success again! (See Figure 17.)

By the time I was finally done, I had stayed an extra four to five hours past my shift. But I left feeling good—two young dogs helped, two families relieved, and two cases that had stumped other clinics solved by my team.

It was the perfect reminder of why we do what we do, and how sometimes… a little wet meat and a screw can turn around even the toughest week.

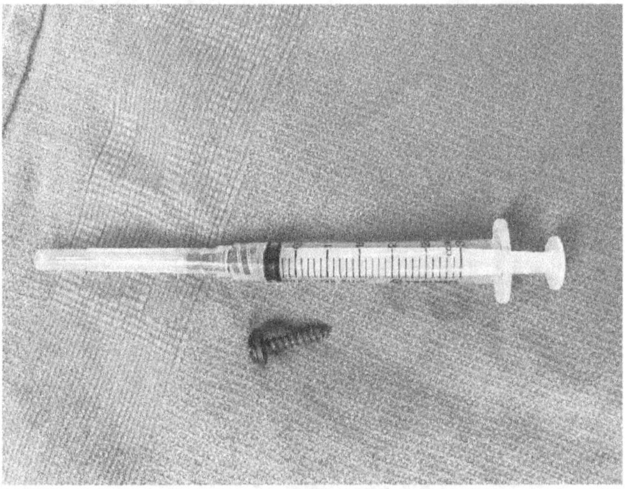

Figures 17

Chapter 10

Managing Mason's mayhem

Mason was a sweet, excitable boxer mix with one very bad habit—eating things he absolutely shouldn't. Over just six months, we saw him about ten times for various ingestions. Sometimes it was toxins like Advil (ibuprofen) or cigarette butts. Other times it was potential foreign bodies, like underwear or pieces of a collar.

Fortunately, Mason was usually easy to treat, and his owners were always understanding about how a veterinary ER works. Most of the time, we could successfully decontaminate him or empty his stomach using an injection of apomorphine. Despite its name, apomorphine isn't a pain medication—it's an extremely effective drug for inducing vomiting in dogs, something we use daily in the ER. It works over 95% of the time to make dogs vomit, but it isn't always completely successful at eliminating a toxin or retrieving a foreign object. On average, we can remove 70% or more of a dog's stomach contents, but if the toxin has already been absorbed, additional treatment—like IV fluids and organ function monitoring—is often needed. For foreign bodies, we have about a 70–80% success rate if the object is still in the stomach. If it's already in the intestines, we don't induce vomiting at all.

Inducing vomiting is not without risks, which is why we never recommend doing it at home. A dog can experience a vaso-vagal response, leading to a sudden drop in heart rate and fainting. They can aspirate vomit into their lungs or choke on the material. In a veterinary hospital, we're equipped to manage these complications immediately.

While there are home remedies—like salt water or hydrogen peroxide—we only recommend them when no other option is available. Salt can dangerously raise blood sodium levels, and hydrogen peroxide almost always causes stomach or esophageal ulcerations.

For Mason, apomorphine worked nearly every time—until one memorable day. He came in after eating something he shouldn't have, but he'd also recently scarfed down a large meal. When we induced vomiting, the sheer amount of material coming up was impressive—and a little alarming. He nearly aspirated because, for some reason, Mason didn't bother to open his mouth. The result looked like something out of a Play-Doh Fun Factory, with vomit squeezing out between his teeth and the sides of his cheeks (see Figure 18). We laughed—poor Mason—but we also had oxygen, suction, and intubation equipment on standby just in case.

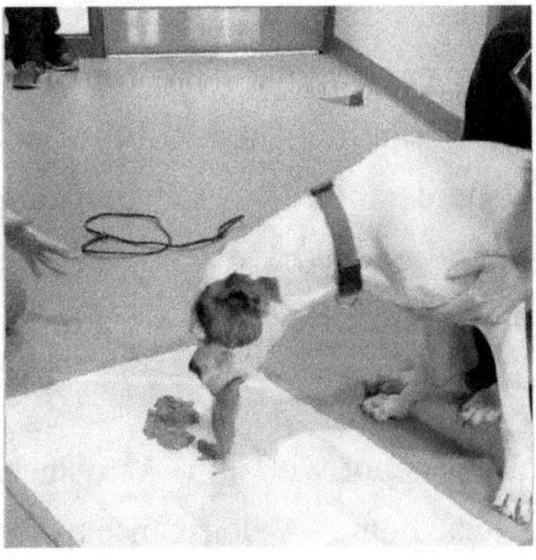

Figures 18

This visit had one more surprise in store. His owners weren't entirely sure what he'd eaten, but they'd seen him slurp up a dark object along with other things from the ground. An X-ray confirmed his stomach was packed with food (most of which we saw squeeze out of his cheeks), but no obvious foreign material came up during vomiting.

Afterwards, while Mason was still a bit sedated from the medication, we finished his exam—including a rectal exam. That's when we felt something large and firm. With a little lubrication, gentle coaxing, and the limited sedation window we had, we managed to pull out an entire pine cone. Yes—an actual, full-size pine cone. I still can't believe it made it all the way through his gastrointestinal tract without causing serious damage. (Figure 19 has the photographic proof.)

Poor Mason went home with some supportive care and recovered well… until, about a month later, we saw him again for yet another round of "things Mason should not eat."

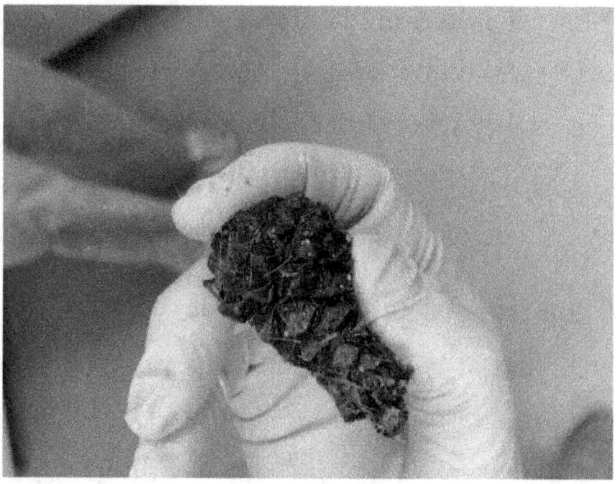

Figures 19

Chapter 11

Hallowen (that's not a typo)

This one actually comes from my wife, who at the time was also working as an ER veterinarian. Before I get to the Labrador, there's a term in veterinary medicine we (probably inappropriately) call "vetcest"—a mash-up of "veterinarian" and "incest." Don't worry, there's no actual incest involved. It's just that veterinarians tend to pair up with others in the veterinary field. The hospital where I spent most of my career had over thirty doctors—mostly ER vets and specialists—and a surprising number were married to other veterinarians. It's not limited to vets, either; technicians and other staff often end up together. Sometimes they work at the same hospital, as my wife and I did for a year, and sometimes at different clinics.

It makes sense. We share a passion for animal care, we spend years in veterinary school together, and once we're working, most of our free time is swallowed by the job. We also meet our partners during the life stage when many people are forming long-term relationships. And when you've had a long day, it's nice not to have to explain why a case was so frustrating—your partner just gets it.

Anyway, that long detour was just to say: my wife is also a veterinarian. We met at work (no shock there) when she was still in emergency medicine, before she decided it wasn't the long-term path for her. After a short break planning our wedding, she found her true niche in veterinary rehabilitation—helping animals with chronic pain or mobility issues from neurological and orthopedic problems. She's become an expert in that field, using therapies like acupuncture, underwater treadmill, and laser treatments. She's helped our own dogs through pain, and it's been amazing to see her improve so many lives.

But back to the Labrador.

While my wife was on duty as an ER doctor, she got a call about a dog who had eaten some gel clings—those colorful, seasonal decorations people stick to windows. They're nontoxic, so the usual protocol is an injection of apomorphine and then removing them via vomiting. This particular Labrador was otherwise healthy, so my wife induced vomiting. The dog brought up food mixed with black and orange gel cling pieces.

When the owners first called, they told us simply, "She ate the window gel clings." We asked for more details—size, shape, what they looked like—and they replied, "How many letters are in 'Happy Halloween'?" That got a laugh. We asked if the clings had been chewed up or swallowed whole. "She's the type to swallow them whole," they said, "but we're not sure."

The vomiting worked beautifully. As is tradition, the team began picking through the pile (yes, we really do that—and yes, it's oddly satisfying). Among the kibble were orange, black, and purple gel letters. Piece by piece, they reassembled most of the phrase "HALLOWEN"—missing only the second "E"—plus two small gel-cling bats. The owners confirmed they'd been missing that "E" and the bats before the dog's snack. (See Figure 20.)

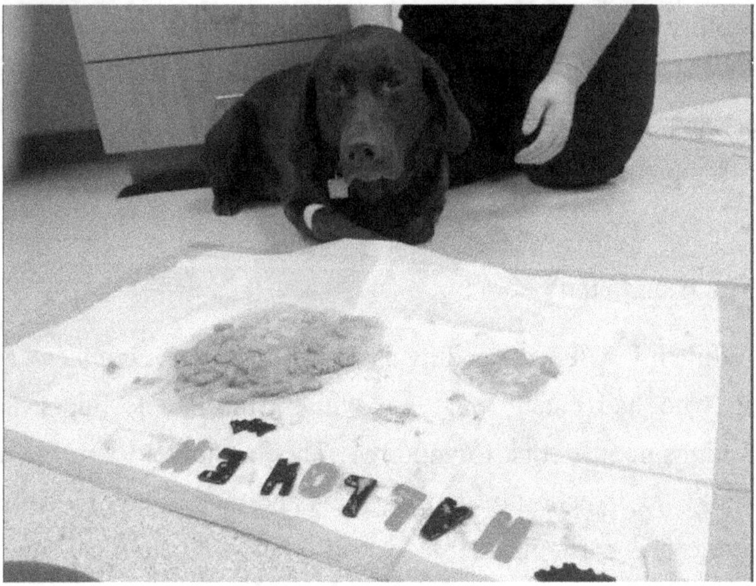

Figures 20

And then came the moment we always ask: “Do you want it back?” Most owners, as these did, politely decline when faced with items fresh from their dog’s stomach.

Still, my wife told them it was one of those stories she’d remember forever. Sometimes owners appreciate hearing that; sometimes, not so much. In this case, the owners didn’t seem impressed, but we were still thrilled the dog was fine—and amused by the circumstances.

Here’s the final twist. My wife loves holiday decorations. When her team was cleaning up, she said, “Wait—these weren’t chewed, they were swallowed whole… anyone want them?” The answer was a resounding no. Undeterred, she washed them thoroughly and stuck them on a treatment room window for the team to enjoy through the season. She even filled in the missing "E" with a washable Sharpie. And that's how "Happy Hallowen" lived on.

Chapter 12

How many of WHAT did you eat?!?!

Dogs eat tampons. A lot. I've lost count of how many cases I've seen—but here's the kicker: they're never new, still-in-the-wrapper tampons. Always used ones. Always.

About six months before writing this, I took a dog to surgery for exactly that. The tampons were lodged in her stomach and intestines, so I had to cut into the stomach and two separate sections of intestine to remove them all—eight in total. Thank goodness for surgical gloves. When I called the owner to share what we found, she was mortified, apologizing that I had to remove them. I assured her it was nothing to be embarrassed about—it happens, and it's part of my job. I was just glad we got to her dog in time. Of course, here I am writing about it, so maybe I enjoyed the story a little too.

I've even been on the other side of the table. Our own new pup once raided the bathroom trash, and we had to rush her to the hospital to induce vomiting. We learned our lesson—our house now boasts large, heavy, dog-proof trash cans. Over the years, I've had to take two of my own dogs to surgery for foreign body obstructions, so I know firsthand how stressful these cases can be.

This particular story stars a golden doodle who showed up at our hospital several hours after getting into the bathroom trash while her owners were out to dinner and a show. They didn't know exactly what had been in there, but the bin had been full—and now it wasn't.

Fortunately, they got her in quickly enough that everything was likely still in the stomach, so we could induce vomiting. It's never a guarantee we'll empty the stomach completely, but it usually works well. We drew up a small syringe of apomorphine and injected it. First came a little drooling, then the lip curl of nausea, then stomach contractions—ten or twelve before the first attempt, followed by five or six rounds of vomiting.

Five of us gathered to watch. (Yes, we watch. There's something strangely entertaining about it.) One staff member stayed ready in case of complications. The first heave produced nothing, and we were briefly disappointed. But on the second contraction—oh my. "Wow!" and "Oh my God!" rang through the treatment area. Out came a massive pile of tampons, pads, and other assorted bathroom trash. Then it happened again. And again. And again.

By the end, the dog had produced five or six piles, each smaller than the last. She sat proudly beside the final heap, captured in a photo (Figure 21). Final count: forty-eight tampons, plus a few pads. Truly impressive.

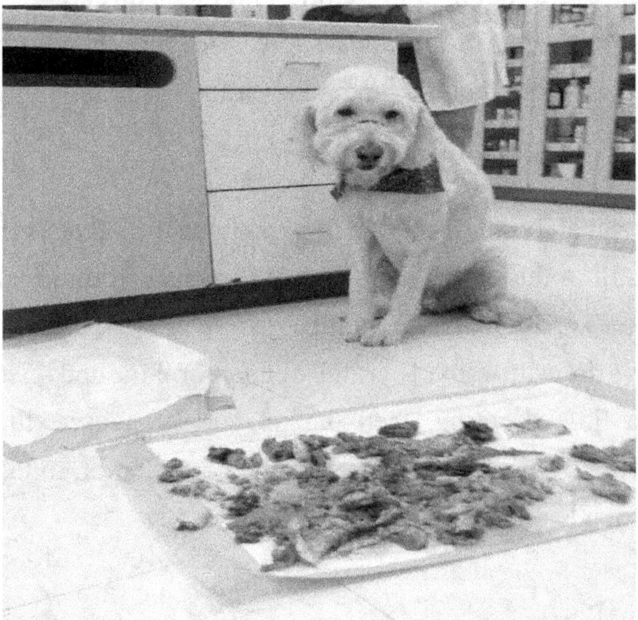

Figures 21

Section 3

Survival

Chapter 1

Common sense escapes some people

At the emergency clinic, we get phone calls every single day from pet owners asking what to do in all kinds of situations. Most of the time, we know exactly how to guide them. Other times, it's not so clear—or it's something none of us have ever seen before. The good news? At least they're calling the right people. Asking your vet is always better than asking the internet. The bad news? Sometimes they call at the least convenient times…but I'll get to that.

Most questions fall into predictable categories:

- **"My dog is vomiting, should I bring him in?"** (Usually yes, especially if he's acting lethargic.)
- **"My dog ate X, Y, or Z. What should I do?"** (Could be chocolate, medication, socks—sometimes dangerous, sometimes not. If we don't know, we call poison control.)
- **"My dog was supposed to give birth, but nothing's happening. What should I do?"**
- **"My pet is limping, can I give it some pain medication?"**
- **"I accidentally gave two doses of the same medication. What now?"**

The list goes on.

Some cases sound trivial but aren't. For example: "My cat is just hanging out in the litterbox, but not doing much." Owners sometimes brush that off. In reality, if it's a male cat, this could be a **life-threatening urinary obstruction**.

Here's why: male cats have tiny urethras (1–2 mm wide). It doesn't take much—crystals, mucus plugs, inflammatory debris—to block that tube. Once urine can't get out, waste products build up in the blood. The most dangerous is potassium. High potassium can slow and then completely stop the heart within hours. Symptoms vary: some cats look painful, some vomit, others are just lethargic. Which is why our standard advice is: *"If you're worried enough to call, we're worried enough to recommend you come in."*

And then there are the calls that leave us face-palming. Here are some real ones:

- **Owner:** "My dog just gave birth. While chewing off the umbilical cord, she pulled too hard, and now some intestines are coming out. That can probably wait until morning, right?"
  Us: "Wait…INTES-TINES? No. Get here *now.*"
  (Sometimes the owner still says, "We'll wait and see." Cue us banging our heads on the desk.)
- **Owner:** "My cat was limping, so I gave him Tylenol. Then I Googled it and saw it's toxic. What should I do?"
  Us: "Bring him in immediately. Even one pill can kill a cat."
  (If only they had called first…)

- **Owner:** "My dog has been shaking uncontrollably for two hours. I think he's seizing. He's not responsive anymore. Should I bring him in?"
  Us: "YES. NOW."

- **Owner:** "My dog seems to be having trouble breathing. I tried putting him in the bathroom with a hot shower running, then took him for a long walk, but he's still struggling. What should I do?"
  Us (trying not to scream): "Difficulty breathing is *always* an emergency. Get him in."

- **Owner:** "My dog was hit by a car. He walked fine at first, but now he's not moving and has blood coming from his eye and ear. Do you think I should bring him in?"
  Us: "Yes. Immediately. Please."

And then there's the classic: owners who feed their dog right after it vomits. If you've ever been nauseated yourself, what's the first thing you wanted to do? I'll bet it wasn't to sit down to a steak dinner. Let the stomach rest!

So here's my plea: If you're not sure, call us. We'll give you honest advice. Don't waste time Googling—or worse, asking AI that doesn't know your pet. Some internet info is solid, but a lot isn't. When in doubt, just call. We'll help.

Chapter 2

Clothing is always coming off at the vet hospital

I'm not always sure what prompts people to take off their clothes, but there are countless instances of clothing—or the lack thereof—becoming an unexpected feature of the veterinary ER. Some of these occasions are more disturbing than others. Don't worry, I don't have any pictures of clients for this chapter.

I can come up with a few reasons why clothes might come off in the veterinary ER, but personally, I find it inappropriate to remove clothing in public. So why do others feel it's fine at a vet hospital? I'm not entirely sure, but some clarification is definitely needed.

There are really two main scenarios: clients who arrive missing clothing, and those whose clothes come off during their visit. Starting with the first—why would someone show up at a veterinary hospital partially dressed? Usually, it's because something drastic happened quickly, and in that moment of panic, the owner decided that speed was more important than being fully clothed. Honestly, the only reason we don't see completely naked clients is simply that most people are already wearing at least a base layer of clothing most of the time. Think about it: how often are you truly naked? In the shower, maybe while changing, or while sleeping—unless you're a dedicated nudist, it's rare. So the odds are in our favor that even in a hurry, people show up wearing at least *something.*

Still, I can see how emergencies catch people off guard. I had a close call myself not long ago. I was about to hop in the shower when I heard our dogs harassing the cat. Normally, the cat is kept separate, but that day he (the cat) had snuck upstairs and hid under the bed. The dogs followed me upstairs as part of my morning routine, and before I'd finished disrobing, chaos erupted. The dogs lunged under the bed, the cat leapt over my shoulder, and in the process, one of those crazy animals knocked over a floor lamp, smashing it into shards across the floor. Luckily, no one was hurt, but in that moment, if someone had been bleeding badly, I could easily imagine rushing out the door before putting all my clothes back on. That said, full nudity in public? Not going to happen for me. Pants and a shirt would go back on no matter what. Not everyone makes that choice, though.

Most often, the missing items are smaller things—shoes, jackets, or sometimes shirts (usually men's). For the most part, pants and shirts remain, and thank goodness for that. We don't officially have a "no shirt, no shoes, no service" rule in veterinary medicine, but maybe we should. Or at least keep a spare set of scrubs in the back for clients who arrive underdressed.

Occasionally, things escalate. Sometimes undergarments are skipped—often for understandable medical or personal reasons. Honestly, most of the time I don't notice or care. But occasionally, it becomes impossible *not* to notice.

I'll never forget one particular case. An older, rather obese client rushed in because her male cat had a urinary obstruction. As I've explained before, this is a common but serious emergency in cats, so when she called, we urged her to come right away. She took that to heart—so much so that she skipped a few crucial steps of getting dressed.

When she arrived, she was wearing an oversized, dirty white T-shirt riddled with holes—with some of those holes placed in rather unfortunate locations. She was also without a bra. After examining her cat and forming a treatment plan, I went to the lobby to meet her. She shuffled in with the help of a cane, her stride causing her chest and midsection to swing rhythmically like a pendulum. Between her gait, the lack of undergarments, and the strategically placed holes in her shirt, let's just say things became more…animated than I would have liked. Unfortunately, I had chosen to sit while she approached, which meant everything was at eye level. Oh boy!

It's not often that we have "nip slips" in the veterinary clinic, but that day, they happened repeatedly—in the middle of our lobby, no less. Still, professionalism prevailed. I kept my focus on her cat, explaining that he would need pain medication, sedation, and both a urinary catheter and an IV catheter to relieve his obstruction. Meanwhile, I did my best to ignore the unintended show.

However, after noticing I had used the word *catheter* repeatedly, she went on to explain how she had once been hospitalized in the recent past and needed a catheter herself. She proceeded to tell me in detail how difficult it was for the medical staff to pass a urinary catheter in her. I can appreciate this, as it's harder to pass urinary catheters in female veterinary species, and it's a challenging skill to master—much more difficult in a female than in a male. Maybe I should also point out that I didn't really ask for these details, but this is just another thing that people often do with veterinarians, a habit so common it has its own name: the "overshare."

She continued in vivid detail: "I remember, they were having such a difficult time. There were two or three people digging around *"down there"*, trying to get the catheter in, and then they had to call the senior nurse, as she was the only one who was able to get the urinary catheter in." It was quite a descriptive story for me that day… and not one I really needed to hear.

As with many of the stories in this collection, it's very common for people to digress in their storytelling about their pets. I was trying to talk about the treatment her cat needed, and she was telling me about the time she had to get a urinary catheter. Really, those things are hardly related, but people always want to share their story.

I'm sure the next words out of my mouth were, "Anyway… back to your cat," as I tried to steer the conversation back to the problem at hand.

We ended up treating her cat. He did very well and went home within a day or two feeling just fine, with a change in diet to help prevent urinary crystals we found in his urine—a contributing factor to the urinary obstruction he had. All of us at the clinic wanted to prevent that urinary obstruction from occurring again in that particular cat, and for more than one reason!

So, the second reason why clothing is sometimes missing at the veterinary hospital: people, for various reasons, voluntarily disrobe. "Why?" you might ask. Well, let's get into that.

As we all know, dogs and cats in particular have incredibly keen senses of smell, far sharper than our silly human noses. And most of us also know that certain smells can be closely tied to memories. Smell is a powerful trigger, capable of bringing back moments in vivid detail—sometimes good, sometimes bad.

For example, you might remember what it smelled like when you came home from school as a child and someone was baking cookies. Or you might recall the comforting smell of your own house or bedroom. Maybe the smell of freshly cut grass brings back summer memories. The list goes on.

We can all agree that animals likely remember smells as well. Their "mental smell vault" is probably far richer than ours, thanks to their heightened olfactory ability. The only problem is, we don't know what those smells bring to mind for them. I'm sure our pets love our smell—we're the ones who feed them and love them—but does that smell translate into a sense of comfort when they're away from home, or into memories of their beloved family? Nobody really knows.

Still, many clients believe that leaving something that smells of home—or more specifically of themselves—must be comforting when their pet is hospitalized and away from their "pack." Maybe it is, maybe it isn't. It's hard to say for sure.

Despite this belief, most owners don't remember to bring their dog's blanket, toy, or piece of clothing to leave with them during a hospital stay. Understandably so—I wouldn't remember either. And so, this is the second most common reason people remove clothing in the veterinary clinic: to leave something with their pet that smells like them.

These items vary, but the most common things I've seen are socks and shirts. Yes, people are willing to strip off clothing—sometimes marching around shirtless (both men and women!)—to make sure their pet has something familiar. And while that smell is likely comforting to their pet, I'll be honest: it's not comforting for me or my coworkers.

One thing that is rather unsettling for the staff is that those "comfort items," if they smell strongly enough to be familiar to the animal, are usually sweaty, dirty, and full of bacteria and skin cells. That's what body odor is! And while we all love our pets and our staff loves getting close to patients too, we don't exactly enjoy having someone's sweaty socks lying around the clinic.

On a secondary note, you should know that veterinary hospitals do a *lot* of laundry. Any cloth material that goes in a kennel with a pet is likely to get soiled during their stay. We do take pets outside regularly, but accidents happen—sometimes diarrhea, sometimes bloody discharge, sometimes just plain excessive urination. We change kennel blankets constantly. We always want our patients to have clean bedding, so we warn owners that anything left with their pet will be washed, and sometimes things get lost in the laundry—never to be seen again. Just like socks in your dryer at home, things vanish, and sometimes items get mixed up because they look alike.

So if it's a favorite shirt or a special blanket from home, it's probably best to take it back with you. Otherwise, it may disappear into the great abyss of vet clinic laundry.

The third, final, and most disturbing reason clients take off clothing at the veterinary clinic, I think, stems from an episode of

Seinfeld. I looked it up: Season 8, Episode 10. For those of you who know the characters, Jerry's eccentric neighbor Cosmo Kramer developed a nagging cough one day. Around the same time, he became acquainted with a dog named Smuckers, who had a similar cough. Kramer took the dog to the vet, figuring they had the same condition.

Kramer declared, "Oh, I'll take a vet over an MD any day. They've got to be able to cure a lizard, a chicken, a pig, a frog—" (snapping his fingers with each species) "—all on the same day."

Well, that part is true. Veterinarians are proud of the fact that we often treat multiple species in the same day. Over the years, I've seen plenty of vet-themed gifts—t-shirts, mugs, etc.—with the slogan: *Real doctors treat more than one species.* It's something unique about our profession, and something many of us (myself included) take pride in. Another common joke among veterinarians is that it's statistically harder to get into veterinary school than medical school. By that logic, we joke that the "average veterinarian" is smarter than the "average MD" Obviously, that's not really true, as there are good and bad practitioners in both professions, and success involves a lot of qualities you can't measure on paper.

Anyway, back to *Seinfeld.* Kramer began taking the same medication prescribed to Smuckers, and before long, he started developing dog-like behaviors and mannerisms. Classic sitcom absurdity, of course. But as any reasonable person should know, taking medication prescribed for your pet is *never* recommended. Please don't ever take your dog's medication. And while we're at it, please don't give your pet human medication either. Even if some drugs overlap well between species, many are quite different—and the dosage difference between species can be drastic, making many medications unsafe for pets.

I've wandered a bit in the telling for this story, but back to the final reason why people take their clothes off at the veterinary hospital: sometimes clients are a little *too* trusting of their veterinarian. When their dog is suffering from something, they see it as a good opportunity to ask, "While I'm here, could you look at this too?" That's when the client proceeds to lift their shirt, pull down their pants, or otherwise start undressing to show me their own affliction.

I get it, there are actually some potential advantages to asking a veterinarian about your own illness. Veterinarians are far more likely to be aware of common zoonotic diseases (diseases that can be transmitted from animals to people or vice versa). Sometimes, we do need to inform clients that transmission to humans is possible. Examples of zoonotic diseases include rabies, leptospirosis, and ringworm.

However, at the same time, most of us in the veterinary profession find human beings a little bit gross (at least compared to our animal friends), and we are by no means legally able to diagnose or treat people—that is the job of an MD. It's perfectly appropriate to disrobe when instructed at your own primary care physician's office, as it's often necessary for a physical exam. However, disrobing at the veterinary hospital so you can speak to a veterinarian about a human problem is almost never appropriate!

I have had several clients take their clothing off to show me personal skin lesions, whether or not they looked similar to what was going on with their pet. Some simply lifted a shirt or pulled up a pant leg, which was not a big deal. Others, however, have taken their shirts off completely or dropped their trousers and asked me, "While I'm here, Doctor, would you mind taking a look at this rash I have?"

I usually pause in surprise when asked these questions. My response is generally something along the lines of, "If I think this disease might be transmissible to people, I will let you know. Regardless, I am not an MD and cannot treat you, so please put your pants back on."

Since I cannot show you pictures of the people who have come to the clinic missing clothes, I thought I would end this list of unsettling stories with another anecdote. You see, most people are polite enough to keep their clothes on, but some still want to leave something behind for their pet to smell and, hopefully, find comfort in. And so, I leave you with the only picture I have for this section: a cloth referred to by the owner as "The Stinkies" (Figure 1).

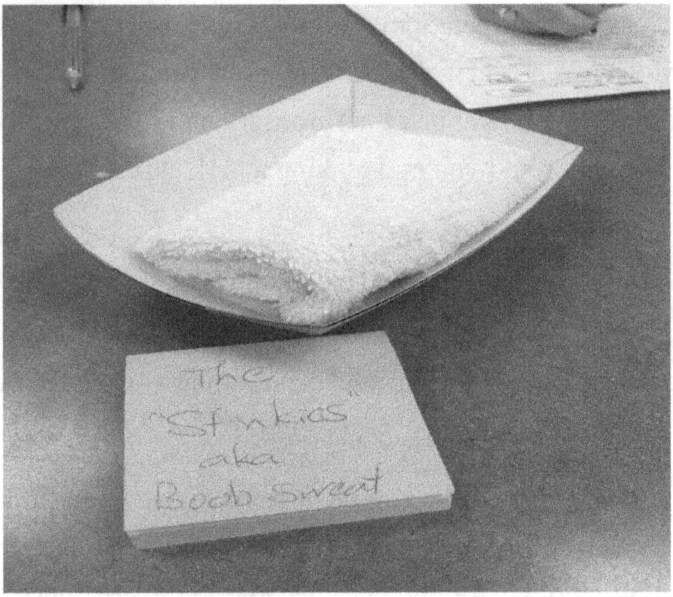

Figure 1

After I had consulted with an owner about her dog, we agreed that it would be best that the dog stay in hospital for treatment—which, by the way, was great news for the pet (and for us) as that dog was going to get all the treatment he needed—I was completely taken aback by what the owner did. The client asked to visit her pet briefly before leaving for the evening. One of our technicians brought the pet to her for a short visit and then returned the dog to the treatment area. On her way out the door, the client asked one of our staff members if we could place a towel in her pet's cage. She called the towel "The Stinkies" for some reason and handed it over to our front desk staff.

The staff member brought this towel to me in the treatment area, and I asked her to explain what "The Stinkies" were—it did not sound very appealing. It turns out the client had taken one of our small exam room hand towels and rubbed it under her breasts to collect sweat, along with her armpits, so it would smell like her. She wanted this towel to stay with her dog.

We did the polite thing and let her dog sniff the towel, but for sanitary reasons, I had to then have it laundered. After that, I could do nothing but sigh and think, "Well, at least she left her clothes on!"

Chapter 3

The zombie apocalypse

The most popular monster in recent popular culture has certainly changed over the years. In just the last two or three decades, zombies, wizards, and vampires have each dominated the scene; this is evidenced by cultural juggernauts such as *Harry Potter*, *The Walking Dead*, and the *Twilight* series. When zombies became so popular, it struck a particular chord with many veterinarians. I've always been a big fan of *The Walking Dead*, and in Season 2, one of the main characters introduced was Hershel Greene, a farmer with veterinary skills. The truth is, a good farmer who has spent a lifetime working with animals can handle a surprising number of situations in a zombie apocalypse—but I guarantee you that no professional would be more useful to your "post-apocalyptic survival team" than a veterinarian.

Shortly after the rise in popularity of *The Walking Dead*, the American Veterinary Medical Association (AVMA) actually published the top five reasons why having a veterinarian on your team would help you survive the zombie apocalypse. Below is a summary of their list, with my own commentary added. The original article can be found on the AVMA website here: https://www.avma.org/public/Health/Pages/you-want-a-veterinarian-on-your-team-in-a-zombie-apocalypse.aspx

Reason #1: Veterinarians have been trained to avoid bites.

This is the most common method of transmission for the zombie-inducing virus—or if not a virus, at least some kind of life-threatening infection. I'm pretty sure it's accepted fact that if you get bitten by a zombie, you're done for. And while plenty of people have some experience restraining animals—farmhands, groomers, or anyone who's given a reluctant dog a bath—in veterinary school we are specifically trained not only how to restrain a wide variety of species, but also how to avoid bite injuries. These lessons often begin in our first or second year of veterinary school during hands-on labs, where we work in pairs or small groups learning both herd management and individual animal restraint. In a post-apocalyptic zombie world, everyone would eventually figure out basic zombie behavior, but veterinarians would likely be quick studies on how to restrain zombies—individually and in groups (herds or hordes). On a daily basis, veterinary staff develop quick reflexes to dodge bites, scratches, and kicks—especially from lightning-fast cats. You'd be surprised how quickly a sugar glider can move, too! These skills would easily translate into avoiding zombies, prolonging our survival and allowing us to teach others how to do the same.

Reason #2: Medical training.

Veterinarians are trained to handle a wide variety of medical situations—everything from infections to broken bones, from anesthesia to wound care. More importantly, we've learned how to do all this when options and resources are limited. Ingenuity is a core skill for us. We practice it constantly: whether working in developing countries, managing during drug shortages, dealing with owner financial limitations, or simply making due, transforming a barn with no electricity into a make-shift surgical suite. During the COVID-19 pandemic, for example, veterinarians were required to stay open but had no access to protective equipment, which was reallocated to human hospitals. So, we made our own. My wife and I built face shields from pool noodles, plastic sheets, and elastic bands. Staff (and my mom!) sewed cloth masks until supplies became available again. In a post-apocalyptic world, equipment like anesthetic monitors, suture, or bandage materials would likely be scarce or non-existent. But don't worry—many veterinarians already know how to perform surgery in poor lighting, bad ventilation, and unpredictable conditions. We are used to training individuals with little to no medical background, like farmhands, to assist us effectively. Unlike a human surgeon—who might complain about the lack of resources—we already know how to adapt, improvise, and work with whatever we have. OK, so we aren't trained to treat humans, but we are trained to treat *every other species on the planet*. That counts for something when it comes to bite wounds, infections, and trauma care.

Reason #3: Animal husbandry and survival skills.

In a zombie apocalypse, society would quickly regress into a pre-industrial state. Indoor plumbing, electricity, and grocery stores would disappear. Farming—both crops and livestock—would become the backbone of survival. And who better to help than veterinarians? Caring for animals, whether pets, livestock, or working animals, is what we do. Where else would horsepower come from if petroleum products ran out? Horses. And who knows how to keep them healthy and useful? Us. Veterinarians could ensure animals remain fit for work, for food, and for companionship, and we would practice herd health to keep communities thriving. This one doesn't even need debate—it's literally our job description.

Reason #4: Food safety.

Veterinarians are trained in the health and management of all food-producing species—pigs, chickens, cattle, and more. Our education covers husbandry, disease development, foodborne illness, humane slaughter, and food processing. We also know how to properly store food to prevent contamination and waste. In a post-apocalyptic world, refrigeration and grocery stores would be gone. Veterinarians could ensure the food supply remains safe, nutritious, and sustainable. Whether it's milk, eggs, meat, or even leather, we'd make sure the animals and the food they provide remain safe for people to consume.

Reason #5: Epidemiology and the cure.

Veterinarians study infectious disease more closely than almost any other profession—especially zoonotic diseases, which cross between animals and humans. If there were any chance of identifying the cause of the zombie infection, controlling its spread, and—dare I say—developing a cure, veterinarians would be essential to the effort. It may sound like an overstatement, but many breakthroughs in vaccines (including COVID-19 vaccines) originated in facilities that began as veterinary research centers. I know this firsthand because I worked at one during my summers in veterinary school. The Vaccine and Infectious Disease Organization (VIDO), located at the University of Saskatchewan, is one such facility, and I even know the current director. So yes, veterinarians could very well help stop the spread—and maybe even save the world.

Chapter 4

Sometimes the funny bone gets hit…at the most inappropriate time

Like any profession, veterinary medicine requires a sense of humor. Those of us working in the hospital often joke about our experiences. To an outsider, our humor might seem inappropriate, but it's never meant that way. We always treat our patients and clients with the utmost respect, but humor is what allows us to keep going. This profession is filled with difficult cases and emotionally draining situations, and when those challenges pile up day after day, a little levity becomes essential. Humor keeps us grounded. Sometimes we go looking for it, and sometimes it finds us.

Every year, when our interns complete their year-long training program, we celebrate their hard work with a dinner. It's a chance to acknowledge the effort they've put into advancing their careers and to send them off with some good memories. For years now, I've tried to bring humor to this event—small gifts, light-hearted jokes about moments from the year, and stories meant to help us all laugh together. I try to be funny without crossing any lines, and sometimes my jokes lands better than others (I have never claimed to be a professional comedian). Maybe someday I'll share those stories in another book, but for now I'll begin with a personal experience—one of those times when humor unexpectedly found me in the veterinary hospital.

To start, I have to touch on one of the most challenging topics in veterinary medicine: euthanasia. For emergency veterinarians and their teams, this is a daily reality, sometimes several times in a single shift. And yet, most veterinary professionals, clients, and support staff can recognize the compassionate side of euthanasia. When an animal's quality of life is gone, when pain and illness have taken over, or when disease has advanced to the point that treatment is no longer humane, euthanasia becomes a final gift. It is not only an option for our animal patients but also an important choice for the families who love them.

These decision to euthanize your pet is never easy, and we understand that. The weight of it became even clearer during the early months of the COVID-19 pandemic in 2020, when physicians faced unimaginable choices about who would receive a ventilator and who would not. In that crisis, human healthcare providers often looked to veterinary medicine for guidance on coping with these kinds of decisions, because we face them regularly. Over the years, our profession has developed coping mechanisms, and many hospitals—including ours—now include veterinary social workers on staff. Their support has become invaluable for both our clients and our medical teams.

Still, euthanasia is emotionally draining, even when we know it is often the kindest choice. There have been days when I've had to euthanize twelve patients in a single shift. That kind of weight stays with you. We try to focus on the positive—relief from suffering, dignity for the animal, peace for the family—but the emotional toll remains. It is one of many reasons why the veterinary profession continues to struggle with high rates of depression and suicide.

Euthanasia is both good and bad. Every one of us has to learn to separate ourselves emotionally from it. When you face so many difficult situations, you try to remind yourself that you're helping the family and ending suffering—but it still takes a toll. I don't think the general public realizes just how often veterinarians participate in euthanasia.

For primary care veterinarians, it can be especially difficult because they've often known the patient for years, sometimes for its entire life. They've cared for the pet through its ups and downs and know the family personally, so when the time comes, it's painful for everyone involved. As an ER veterinarian, I don't usually have that same long-term relationship with the patient or the family. Sometimes that makes it a little easier, but not always. Even meeting a pet and their family for the first time, euthanasia can still hit hard.

For me, there are two particular situations that I find especially difficult, and I know it's because of my own experiences with my own pets. The first is when men cry. The second is when the entire family is present—especially when there are kids in that "tweenage" range. Kids that age often don't know how to process grief. They watch what the adults around them are doing and follow suit, all while managing the emotional rollercoaster of their own stage of life. Euthanasia can be a huge challenge for them, and it's important to be honest and fair during that time.

Many parents struggle with what to tell their children when a beloved pet has to be euthanized. We try to help guide them. For those wondering, the short answer to "What do I tell my kids?" is simple: be honest. Tell them the truth. It's not appropriate to say the pet "went to live on a farm upstate." Death is part of life, and children need the opportunity to experience it in a safe, supported way. It's OK for them to feel emotion and work through it themselves. Younger children may laugh it off and ask for another puppy, middle-aged kids may cry or get angry alongside their parents, and teenagers will go through their own unique process of grief.

Grief itself is fascinating when you understand it. You can recognize the stages, but everyone moves through them in their own order and at their own pace. Eventually, most people reach acceptance, but it's never easy, and it's different every single time.

Other times, euthanasia can bring a sense of release. Families who have fought long, difficult battles alongside their veterinarian may feel relief when the decision is finally made. It's permission to let go, to end the struggle, and to grant their pet peace.

And sometimes, for our own protection, we as veterinarians have to put up emotional barriers. It's not coldness—it's survival. We need to guard ourselves so that we don't break down under the constant weight of loss. Maybe those barriers are a defence mechanism against depression.

Now, I realize this story has gotten heavy, when I originally promised something a little more uplifting. So here it is: every once in a while—very rarely—euthanasia can actually be funny. Humor sometimes surfaces naturally in those moments, and it's often a relief. Families laugh as they remember their pet's quirks, and I've learned hundreds of funny stories that way. But occasionally, the humor comes from the process itself.

This story is one of those times. A first-time client came in with his dog who had bone cancer. The primary care vet had diagnosed it a month earlier, and despite pain medication, the dog was no longer comfortable. The owner knew it was time to say goodbye.

As usual, we placed an IV catheter and gave the owner time to be with his pet. When he was "ready"—though no one is ever truly ready—I came in to explain the process. Typically, we administer a sedative, followed by an overdose of anesthetic. It's painless and peaceful, but the body can sometimes do things as life slips away—muscle twitches, gasps for breath, loss of bladder or bowel control, even eyes remaining open. I always explain this to prepare owners.

This dog's passing began just as expected. He became quiet and limp, stopped breathing, and his heart stopped. I told the owner that his dog had passed. And then, instead of a gasp or a twitch, this very large dog let out a massive, echoing, unbelievably pungent fart.

And it hit me—my funny bone, hard.

I was fighting with every fiber of my being not to laugh. I have never bitten my tongue harder in my life. My eyes filled with tears, which the owner interpreted as compassion for his loss. In truth, I was about to burst.

I quickly excused myself, ran down the hall, shut three doors behind me, and absolutely lost it. I laughed so hard it hurt. My staff looked at me in shock, mouths open, waiting for an explanation. I couldn't even speak. I just waved them off, gasping for a few minutes to collect myself as the laughter poured out.

Finally, I wiped the tears from my eyes, blew my nose, and composed myself enough to return to the room. I apologized for stepping out so quickly. The owner, seeing my watery eyes, thanked me for my compassion. I told him, "I know how hard it is to say goodbye to a family member," and we parted ways.

He was none the wiser, and I was grateful for that. On the outside, I appeared to share his grief. On the inside, I had been holding back the hardest laughter of my career.

Chapter 5

The Decapitation Conversation

Well, I suppose you'll only believe me if I tell you—but sometimes, as part of veterinary medicine, we have to remove the head of a deceased animal. The process is called decapitation.

Before going any further, let me make this clear: this is **only** done after the animal is already deceased, most often after euthanasia. The primary reason is rabies testing. Unfortunately, there is only one way to diagnose rabies: by examining brain tissue under the microscope with a special stain. That means we have to collect fresh brain samples and send them—usually to a government or state lab—for testing.

Getting brain tissue is no easy task. Technically, you could biopsy the brain, but that essentially requires brain surgery, which is expensive, invasive, and unnecessary in these cases. While we do perform brain surgery on animals from time to time—usually for tumors—rabies is different. It's almost always fatal. If an animal has rabies, no amount of treatment will save it.

Here's a sobering fact: tens of thousands of people die annually from rabies. Hard to believe, right? It may feel like this is not true, because in North America, rabies deaths are rare—only a handful occur every few years. That's largely because most pets are vaccinated, reducing human exposure, and because we have broad access to healthcare. When an animal bites someone, the laws are clear: the animal is quarantined and observed, or if euthanized, its brain is submitted for rabies testing. If rabies is even suspected, preventive treatment for the person begins right away. Those of us in high-risk professions—veterinarians, technicians, animal control workers—are also usually vaccinated in advance. The general public is not, both because the risk is so low and because the human vaccine is costly. This is part of our modern healthcare system: prevention, vigilant monitoring and available treatment; these things are not avaialbe in many countries.

Rabies in people is also almost always fatal. As of 2016, only sixteen documented survivors exist worldwide. Sixteen! It's almost unbelievable. I'll get into more detail about rabies in another section of this book, but for now, let's get back to the not-so-glamorous subject of decapitation.

The brain, as you know, is protected inside the skull—a brilliant evolutionary design. Great for preventing injury in a living animal, not so great when you need to collect a fresh sample for rabies testing. When an animal shows abnormal neurological signs or has bitten someone and is euthanized within ten days, laws usually require the head (and therefore the brain) be submitted to the state lab. Rabies is a reportable disease, so veterinarians must comply.

The lab requires that the brain be sent fresh—no preservatives like formalin (which we use for most biopsy samples) and no freezing, since freezing disrupts the cells. Ideally, the brain should be undisturbed. If an inexperienced person tries to extract the brain and damages it, the sample may be ruined. Worse, they could expose themselves or others to the virus in the process. So, the safest and most efficient method is simply to remove the entire head and send it to the lab.

That may sound terrible—and to be honest, it feels terrible doing it at times—but it is always done with respect and always with safety as the top priority. Decapitating the animal and sending the head saves us time, reduces our exposure risk, and ensures the lab gets a usable sample. The state lab technicians are fast, safe, and highly skilled at handling these tissues.

I know it sounds grim, but many of us in the field develop methods to do it as safely and efficiently as possible. Personally, I believe my technique is the best (trust me, it is ☺).

There are several ways to remove a head, but as a busy ER veterinarian, I use the quickest method that balances safety with efficiency. One night, a case like this came up at one of our sister hospitals. A dog had been euthanized, and the head needed to be removed for rabies testing. The attending doctor texted me a question to pass along to one of our technicians, who had recently transferred from that hospital to mine.

Let's just say it was one of those unique text messages that only circulates between veterinary professionals. A screenshot of that exchange is included below (Figure 2).

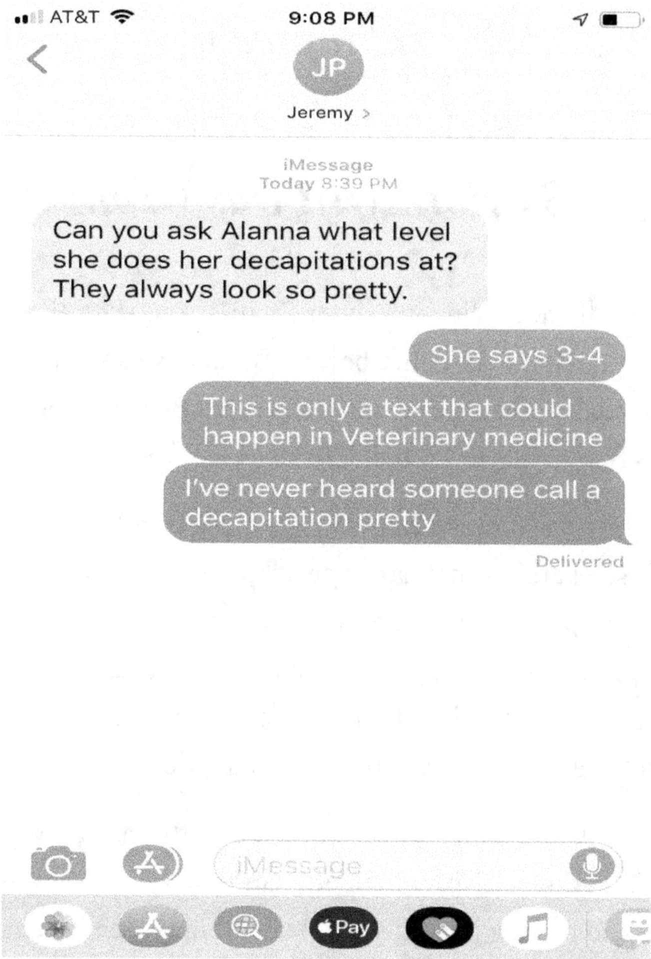
AT&T
9:08 PM
JP
Jeremy >
iMessage
Today 8:39 PM
Can you ask Alanna what level she does her decapitations at? They always look so pretty.
She says 3-4
This is only a text that could happen in Veterinary medicine
I've never heard someone call a decapitation pretty
Delivered
iMessage
Pay

Figure 2

Chapter 6

Taylor Swift was wrong!

Well, there's a line in Taylor Swift's song *Bad Blood* that says, "Band-Aids don't fix bullet holes." But she was wrong—very, very wrong. And honestly, I'm glad she was. Because sometimes all it takes is Band-Aids to fix bullet holes.

A little background might help. Every so often in our veterinary ER, we see patients that have been shot. More often than not, it isn't because the animal was aggressive—it's simply bad luck, being in the wrong place at the wrong time. Sadly, these cases are more common in lower-income neighborhoods, where resources for veterinary care are limited and the animals often pay the price.

There was a time when I wasn't exactly thrilled with our local police department. Now, I should pause here—my brother, brother-in-law, and nephew (and his wife) are all in law enforcement, so I've always been inclined to "back the badge." I respect how hard their job is, especially in recent years. But for a long stretch at our hospital, nearly every gunshot wound in a dog was the result of police encounters. I understand that officers have to protect themselves, especially when executing warrants in dangerous situations, but a little more patience—or animal behavior training—might have spared a lot of pets.

Most of the time, these types of incidents happened during warrant executions. Officers were entering homes where drugs, guns, and money were often present—and often so were dogs. But here's the thing: those dogs were usually just doing what dogs do. They barked to alert their families and protect their pack. Barking doesn't equal aggression. I learned this not only through veterinary training but also through experience with my own Pitbull, Ella. Ella was a therapy dog who visited nursing homes, hospitals, and schools. But if someone had forced their way into our house, she would have barked her head off. "Stranger danger!" she would have shouted in dog language. That's normal behavior. (Figure 3 shows me, many years younger, with Ella on our Delta Society [now called PetPartners] therapy dog badge.)

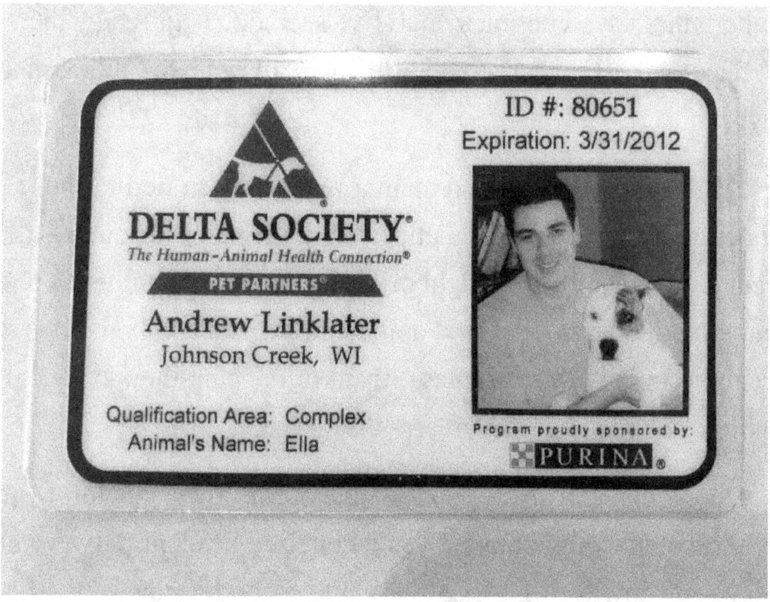

Figure 3

Fortunately, two good things came out of those difficult situations. First, even if a dog was shot, officers almost always brought the animal to us for care. That deserves credit. Second, when we expressed concerns, the police actually listened. Our hospital began offering animal behavior training to officers, and they incorporated it into their programs. Their undercover investigators even started noting whether homes had dogs so that detail could factor into their warrant planning. And it worked: over time, the number of police-related dog injuries we saw dropped significantly. When possible, officers began using non-lethal options like CEWs (conducted energy weapons—Tasers being the common brand name).

CEWs aren't harmless—they disrupt muscles through neuromuscular interference (NMI), which can be painful and, in smaller animals, sometimes fatal. I've seen dogs injured by them. But the fact that officers tried to use them instead of bullets showed progress.

Still, gunshot wounds remain a reality, often tied to those same socioeconomic factors. Sometimes it's neighbor disputes, like the recent case where one neighbor's dog attacked another's, and the second neighbor shot the first dog. Both owners and both dogs ended up in our clinic within minutes—thankfully calm, though we still had to notify police about the firearm discharge.

Here's what I always teach my interns (new doctors): bullets don't travel in straight lines. Even when fired level, gravity eventually pulls them downward. Once they enter a body, however, it's even more unpredictable. Some bullets shatter, some tumble, and tissue density—bone, muscle, organs—redirects their path. They can ricochet around inside a body in ways that make their trajectory nearly impossible to predict.

Television and movies often dramatize the importance of removing bullets; most of the time, the need for bullet removal is fiction. In reality, we often leave them in place. If a bullet is buried deep in muscle or lodged in an organ, surgical removal usually causes more harm than good. Unless it's in a critical spot—like the spinal cord, arteries, or joints—we simply manage the wounds, control pain, and prevent infection. And no, contrary to myth, animals don't die of "lead poisoning" from retained bullets.

Of course, some cases of gunshot wounds are devastating. If a bullet hits a major vessel or vital organ, the animal may not survive. Many die before they even reach us. In other cases, the injuries are so severe that euthanasia is the only humane option. But here's the encouraging part: if the dog is alive by the time they arrive at the ER, chances are good that we can help them with surprisingly minimal care—sometimes just pain relief, cleaning the wounds, bandaging, and antibiotics.

Which brings me back to Taylor Swift's line. I've treated several dogs—two Pitbulls and a Mastiff—that had each been shot multiple times. Their photos (Figures 4–7) look a little gruesome, but keep in mind these dogs were heavily sedated and medicated for pain while we worked on them.

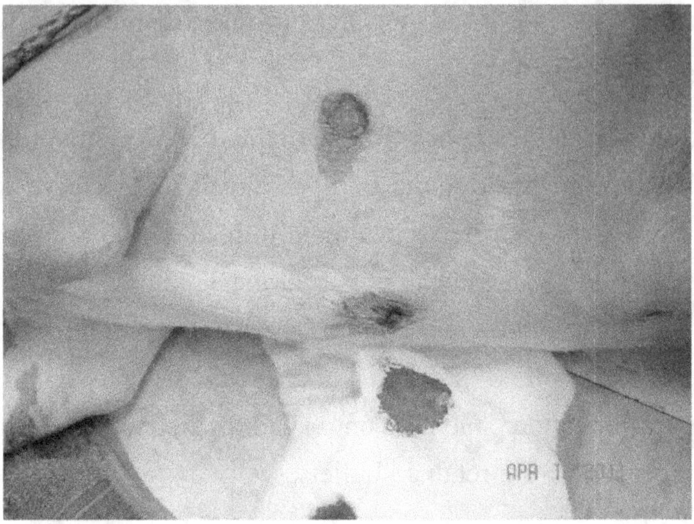

Figure 4

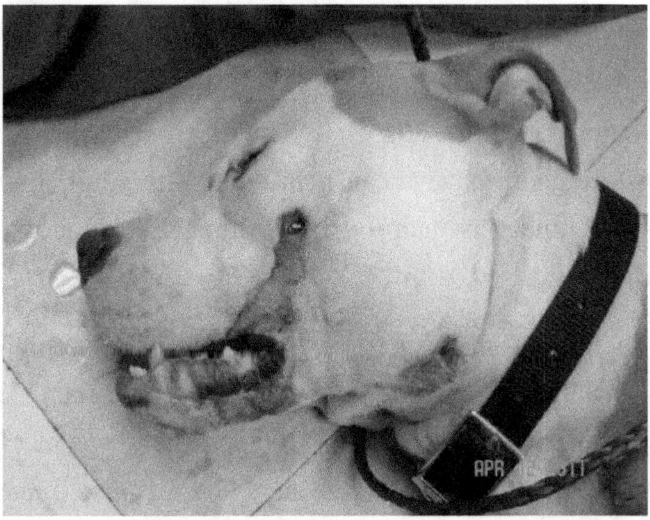

Figure 5

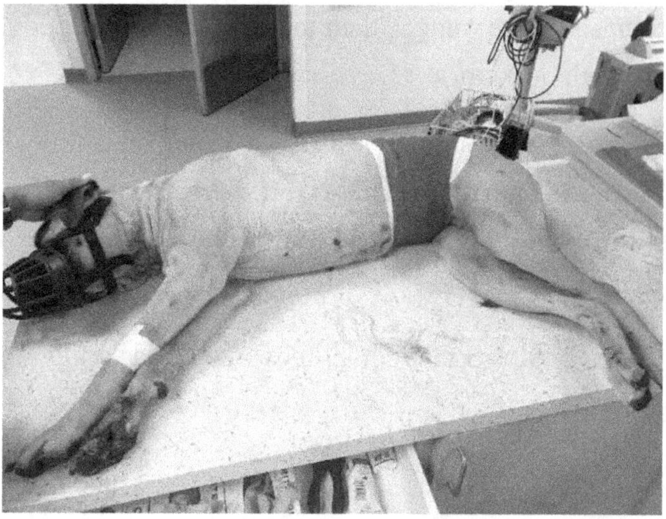

Figure 6

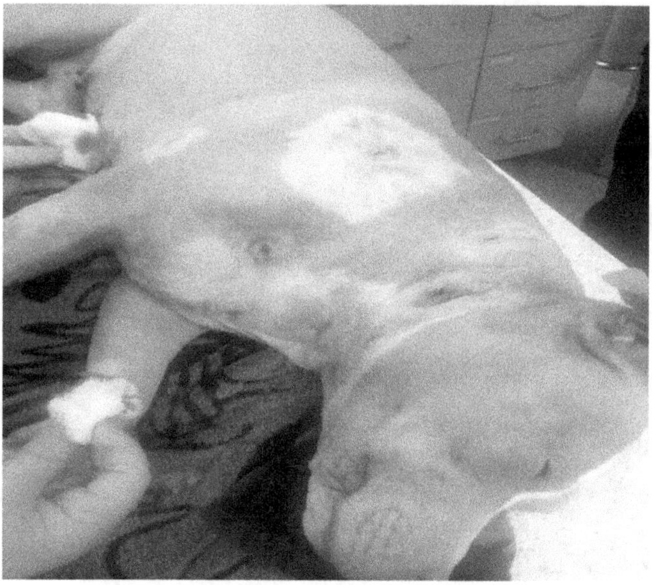

Figure 7

One had entrance wounds in the face and chest. Another was shot in the abdomen. The third, poor guy, had the misfortune of being shot and bitten by another dog at the same time. And yet, despite everything, all three wagged their tails and sought affection when they came through our doors.

Our care was simple: sedation, wound cleaning, bandaging, antibiotics, and pain meds. That was it. Each dog went home the same day, and follow-up reports weeks later showed they were recovering well.

So yes, Taylor Swift, sometimes Band-Aids really do fix bullet holes.

Chapter 7

I should NOT be able to determine your marital status from an x-ray

Every one of us has that "hill we are willing to die on," meaning that there is something we are passionate about in our field, we educate ourselves on it to the fullest extent, we educate our colleagues about practicing the best possible medicine and we generally practice what we preach when it comes to those particular aspects of our job. One of hills I am willing to die on in the veterinary industry, is radiation safety. Quick note of clarification: X-rays are particles of electromagnetic radiation (the literal rays of energy used to take the x-ray 'picture'); a radiograph is the picture created on film (or now, a detector) generated from passing x-rays through tissue onto a detector which you or your doctor look at afterwards.

We are taught early in our careers about the potential dangers of radiation and how we should minimize our exposure to it. Different from when you or I go to the hospital or clinic and have x-rays performed, wherein the x-ray technician steps out of the room or behind leaded glass, in veterinary medicine, the staff often have to restrain the animal in the correct position while standing right next to the animal to perform the radiograph. This means we have increased exposure to those x-rays and potentially increased risk of x-ray related injury if we are not safe.

Our exposure to x-rays is closely monitored with radiation badges, called dosimeters. These badges must be worn when taking these radiographs. We also have personal protective equipment, such as lead aprons, gloves, thyroid collars and more, to protect ourselves from the dangers of chronic radiation exposure.

There are two things you should know about radiation safety for the rest of this story. First, we should ALWAYS be wearing our personal dosimeter and personal protective equipment (PPE) to perform radiographs and second, this PPE is really only designed to protect you from scatter radiation, meaning the x-rays that bounce off the patient or table and fly into the room. The PPE are NOT designed to protect you from the direct x-ray beam. Bottom line of this little lesson is that human body parts should NEVER be seen on a radiograph of an animal. It's kind of a sin in the veterinary world, but you know some people are more diligent about safety than others. If a human body part (usually hands) were *ever* to *accidentally* end up in the radiograph, it surely should be covered by PPE.

Working at a specialty and referral hospital, we get radiographs sent to us on a daily basis from primary care or family veterinarians. And it bugs me to no end when my colleagues perform radiographs and do not wear their personal protective equipment and most importantly, it is dangerous to expose body parts to x-rays unnecessarily. Again, NO HUMAN body part should end up in the x-ray beam and be able to be seen on the radiograph. If this is happening, it means that proper radiation safety is not being practiced and this is a violation of Occupational Health and Safety (OSHA) regulations. Veterinary clinics can have hefty fines imposed if they are found to be not practicing good radiation safety techniques.

So, when the primary care veterinarians send us radiographs and I see human body parts in that radiograph (most of the time it consists of someone's hands), I always call and speak to the senior management team and ask that they speak with their radiation safety officer (RSO), to ensure they are reviewing their radiation safety protocols and following good guidelines. It is a requirement to have an RSO at any hospital that has an x-ray unit.

Sometimes, when hands are in the x-rays, there are rings on those hands, so I can tell if a staff member performing radiographs ismarried or not.... this simply shouldn't happen! Ugh. If no one else can, I will continue to fight this battle! Check out the associated pictures here, Figures 8 and 9. The first one, Figure 8 is a ventrodorsal (or VD) radiograph (taken with the patient lying on its back), the chest is in the middle, and you can clearly see a human hand with rings restraining the patient around the head and neck area. Figure 9 is a little more apparent with human hands straightening out a small dog head for x-rays.

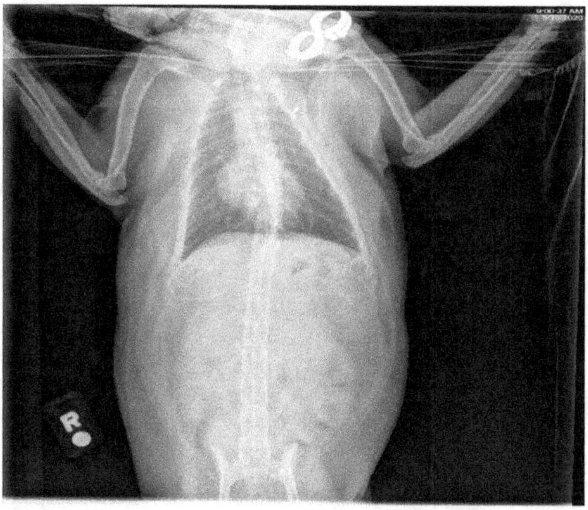

Figure 8

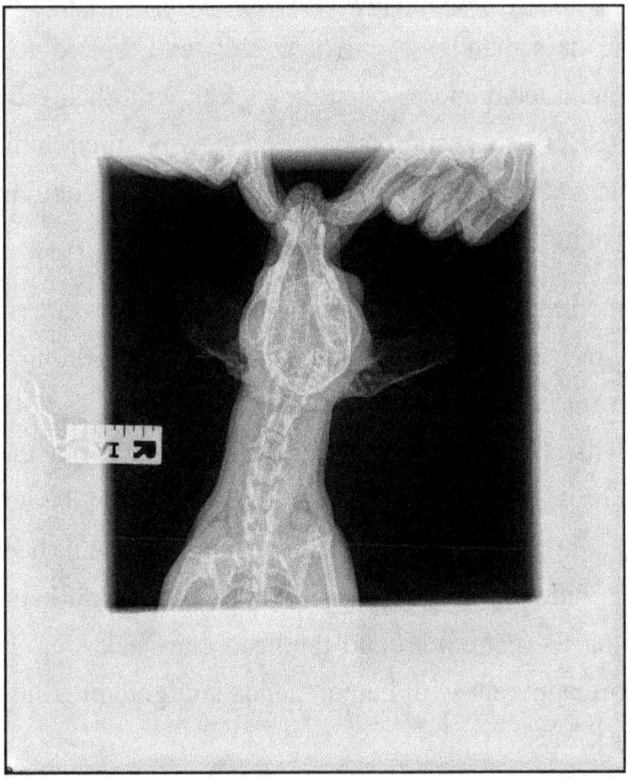

Figure 9

Chapter 8

Did I just pee myself?

It's hard to say how many times someone pees themselves in a veterinary hospital. And while I'm mostly talking about our patients, sometimes the staff has to stop and wonder if it just happened to us too.

With patients, it's expected. They may urinate because of an underlying condition—urinary infections, kidney disease, diabetes—or because they can't get up and move normally after orthopedic surgery. Others urinate because they're lethargic from disease, sedatives, or IV fluids. We anticipate this, so patients are taken outside regularly, their bladders are expressed, or in some cases we place urinary catheters. Even with those precautions, accidents still happen, which means frequent bedding changes are part of our routine.

But when we ask, "Did I just pee myself?" we're really talking about the staff. It's one of those odd little running jokes that helps us get through long, stressful days. Just this past week, several of us had to ask that very question of ourselves.

There are a few reasons why this may happen to the veterinary staff. First and foremost, caffeine. It is the lifeblood of ER medicine, fueling us through nights that never seem to end. And the options are endless: coffee (my choice), energy drinks, soda, 5-hour Energy, chocolate-covered coffee beans, caffeine mints—you name it. Figure 10 shows a couple of my go-to choices on my desk: usually a mug of coffee plus a Dr. Pepper. (I was a fan of the 10-calorie Dr. Pepper Bold, but sadly it's no longer made as everything is zero sugar now.)

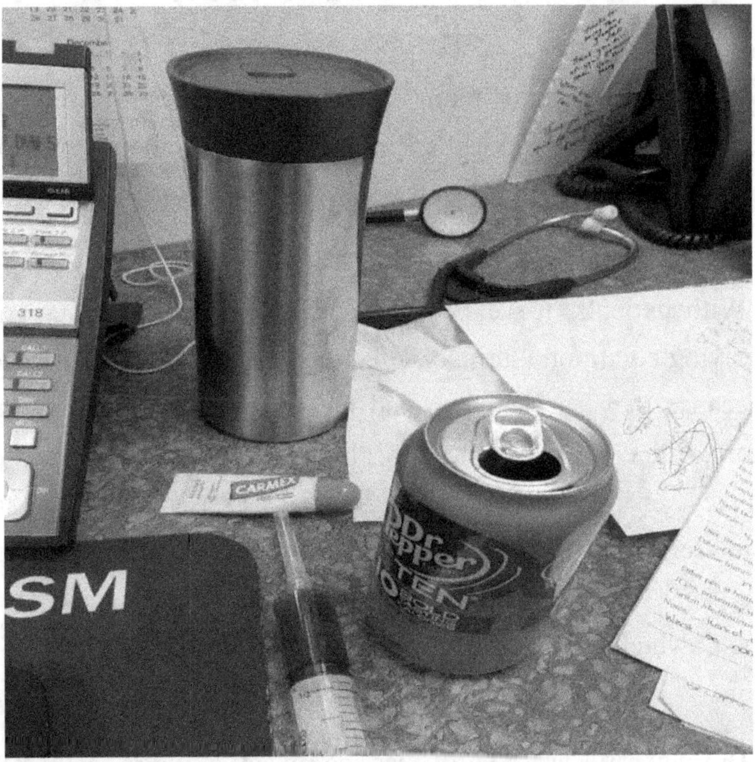

Figure 10

The doctor station—our caffeine headquarters—is also where controlled medications are kept. Right beside my coffee in that picture? A syringe of blue euthanasia solution. Sounds alarming, but it has to stay in our possession until administered, per DEA rules. So yes, I was following protocol.

Second reason: we simply don't have time. ER medicine doesn't exactly accommodate leisurely bathroom breaks. Often, it's the middle of the night before we finally realize we haven't gone in hours, and just as we're about to sneak away, a crisis rolls through the door. Other times we're bouncing between procedures and exam rooms, so focused on our patients that we forget our own basic needs. It isn't that we actually pee ourselves—but on some nights, it feels like we're pushing our limits.

Then there are the moments when we really do end up wet. We work in close quarters with patients: lying beside them, lifting them, carrying them pressed against our scrubs. And of course, animals rarely coordinate bathroom breaks with our schedules. The result? More than a few times, someone is left soaked in urine—definitely not their own. That's why most of us keep a backup set of scrubs at the hospital, and sometimes wish we had two. Figure 11 shows one such moment, captured by my staff for proof.

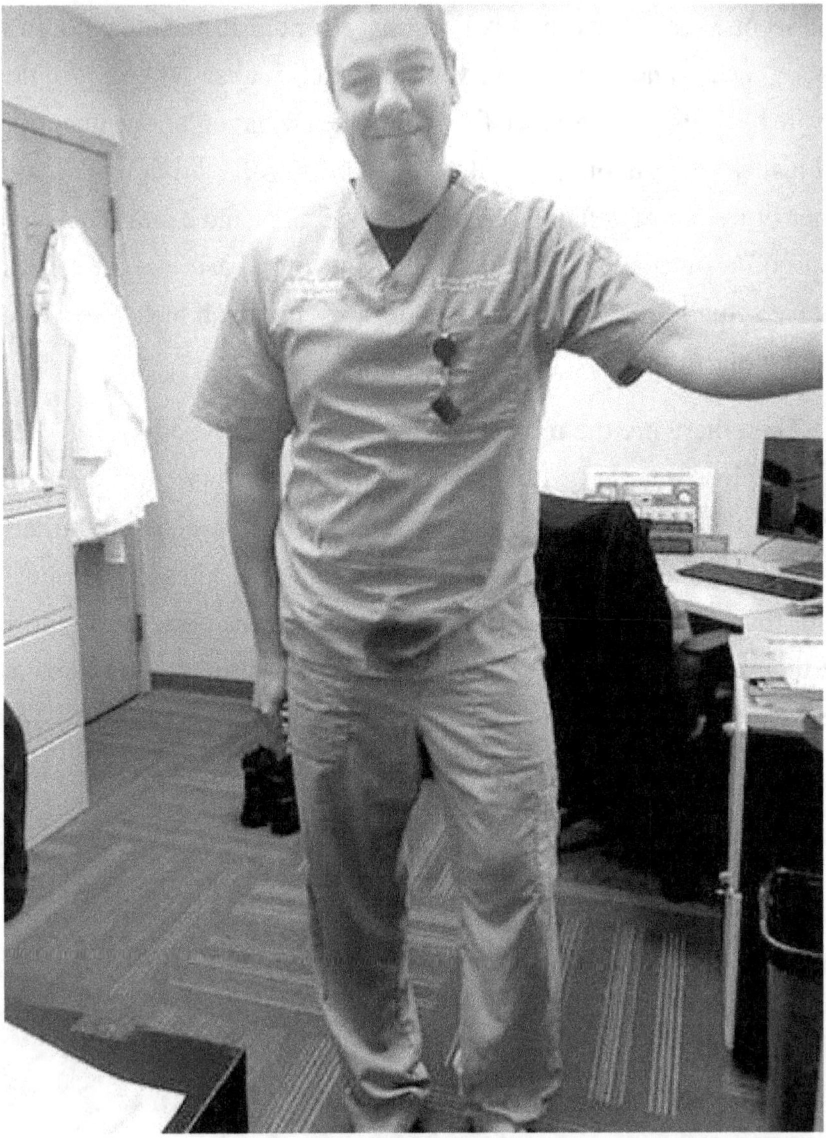

Figure 11

It's always a special feeling to pick up a patient and suddenly realize something warm and wet is spreading across your clothes.

When that happens, our priority is still the patient, which means our own hygiene often gets pushed to the bottom of the list until they're cleaned and comfortable.

And urine isn't the only culprit. Our work tables are the perfect height to meet us at crotch level. Leaning against a wet surface could mean water or shampoo, which isn't so bad—or it could mean something far less pleasant: urine, blood, pus, or diarrhea. A wet sink can be treacherous territory.

Finally, there are the near-miss situations. When I perform echocardiograms or ultrasounds, the patient lies on their side on an elevated table while I slide the probe under them to reach the heart. The skin is shaved, alcohol or gel applied, and an assistant leans over the table to restrain the patient. That setup unfortunately leaves the assistant's crotch exposed between tables. Occasionally, when I reapply alcohol, I miss my target and spray the assistant instead. Oops. At least alcohol is clean, quick-drying, and leaves nothing but a funny story behind.

Chapter 8

Some people, just like some dog breeds, can be screamers

I'd like to say that the majority of our clients don't scream at us, but the truth is, sometimes we have those days when more than one does. I'm not sure what makes someone a screamer—nature versus nurture? In today's world of "Karens" and "I need to speak to the manager" moments, screamers seem to be everywhere. I can tell you this much: in the service industry, screaming gets you nowhere. The louder and more rude a client becomes, the less inclined we are to help. And in veterinary medicine, where we're already overworked and overtired, there are times we'd honestly prefer they take their business to another clinic rather than scream at our staff.

Of course, humans aren't the only screamers. Some dog breeds, just like some people, are naturally vocal. Huskies will howl for hours without tiring. Beagles and hounds bay endlessly. And puppies—oh, puppies!—will squeal at the slightest discomfort, like a vaccination, only to forget seconds later once distracted. Beyond that, vocalization often depends on the dog's mental state. Hyper-excitable breeds, such as Vizslas and Weimaraners, can be particularly noisy (I like to call Weimaraners "whiny-rawners"). Labradors are unpredictable—sometimes quiet, sometimes relentless—but chocolate Labs seem especially prone to whining. Don't get me wrong, I love them all, but when a hospitalized dog whines or "screams" for hours, it's stressful for them and exhausting for us. The causes vary—loneliness, boredom, separation anxiety—and while pain is always a possibility, we aggressively manage pain and use it as a last explanation.

In the hospital, we try a variety of strategies to help these dogs. Spending time with them in their kennel is our favorite (though time-consuming) approach. At my current hospital, we even use special lights that mimic circadian rhythms, and we'll play calming music or videos. Still, the ICU is a busy, stimulating environment—not always the easiest place for patients to rest. When they finally do fall asleep, we work hard to keep them that way: lowering noise, covering kennels with towels to reduce visual stimulation, and sometimes even using earplugs. Yes, you read that right—we keep earplugs at the clinic, originally for screaming pigs (see Section 5), but more often they're for dogs…and occasionally even placed in dogs' ears. You'd be surprised how well it works. When those options aren't enough, we move to what I call "better living through chemistry"—calming medications, given either orally or by injection. It's not just for our sanity, but also for the patients' comfort and recovery.

I should clarify two important points here. First, when I say "screaming," I mean vocalizing—howling, whining, or barking—not literal screams. Second, I know some readers may worry this means patients are in pain. Please know: pain management is our top priority. Our ER and ICU use a validated system called the Composite Modified Pain Scale (CMPS) to carefully assess discomfort. It evaluates vocalization, attention to painful areas, mobility, response to touch, demeanor, and posture, scored from 0 to 24. Any score above 6 means pain relief is administered immediately. Most hospitalized animals actually do well—they're comforted by staff presence, distracted by the activity around them, and often too unwell to behave normally.

But back to the real problem: screaming clients. These are far more frustrating than noisy dogs. Most veterinarians and staff are not formally trained to handle angry, yelling clients. Veterinary schools are improving communication training, and we now offer staff de-escalation workshops, but ultimately there's only so much we can do when someone is intent on screaming.

We do understand that clients are scared, anxious, and heartbroken about their pet's situation in the ER. Many of us have been through it with our own animals. But taking that frustration out on the people trying to help doesn't make sense. Often, clients are polite to the doctor but rude to technicians or front desk staff. Believe me, we notice. And when someone mistreats my team, it affects me too. It's not that we care less for their pet, but trust and civility are essential for effective care. Without mutual respect, communication breaks down, and that hurts the patient most of all.

A common misconception that fuels anger is the cost of veterinary care. Clients assume we order unnecessary tests or treatments for money. That couldn't be further from the truth. In fact, we spend a lot of energy finding ways to minimize costs, because we know finances are a burden—many of us couldn't afford our own recommendations if our pets were sick. Unlike human medicine, veterinary medicine has no government subsidies, insurance mandates, or universal coverage. Costs come directly out of owners' pockets. Even then, veterinary care is priced significantly lower than comparable human care. The reality is, we must charge for services:

hospital expenses, equipment, medications, and most importantly, staff salaries. Add in the fact that most veterinarians graduate with six-figure student loan debt, and it's clear that no one is in this for the money.

For us, it's always about the animals. We took an oath to care for them, and we wouldn't do this job otherwise. But when clients scream, curse, or threaten us, it makes it incredibly difficult to maintain compassion. Would you yell at your dentist, doctor, mechanic, or insurance broker and expect better service? Probably not. Please, don't scream at us. Vent about the situation, cry, even curse the universe for your pet's illness—that's all understandable. But screaming at the staff only strains the relationship, and if that relationship is broken, it's much harder for us to work together toward your pet's best outcome.

Interestingly, screamers come from every background and level of education. Some curse, others lash out physically—at me, at themselves, or even at the walls and furniture. In the next section, I'll share three stories of clients who screamed at me and how I handled it. Some recognized the error of their ways. Others probably left thinking their behavior was perfectly acceptable.

In our hospital, we actually have a code of conduct posted for everyone to see—something we expect both ourselves and our clients to follow. Simply put, if you cannot treat our staff in a civil manner, we would rather have your pet cared for elsewhere. When someone treats me or our team disrespectfully, I usually give them one warning. That way it's clear their behavior has been noticed, they understand how it's affecting communication, and they have an opportunity to improve.

It's not an easy conversation to have when someone is yelling at me, but it often goes something like this: "Mr. Smith, you're screaming and swearing at me. I'm here to help you and your pet, but if you're not willing to communicate in a civil manner, I'm more than happy to help you find another hospital where you may feel more comfortable." In other words, please calm down and talk to us like adults. If the behavior continues after that warning, they can be "fired" as a client. Of course, we'll still help transfer their pet's care to another hospital, because the animal deserves treatment, but sometimes mutual respect is simply not possible.

You may be asking yourself, *"Wait, a veterinary hospital can fire clients?"* Absolutely. While we want to help every patient, we are under no legal obligation to do so. Veterinary medicine is, at its core, a service industry—and a very busy one at that. None of us are willing to tolerate abuse just to do our jobs. On top of that, in order to provide care, we are legally required to have a veterinary-client-patient relationship (VCPR). If that relationship is broken or toxic, we cannot do our jobs effectively, and in those rare cases, we do let clients go.

Thankfully, most people—once the problem is pointed out—recognize they're being uncivil, adjust their behavior, and we move forward. The rare few who feel justified in their hostility are the ones we do not allow back. That doesn't mean we abandon their pet. We still provide medical recommendations and help transition care, but we limit contact with those individuals. Veterinary medicine is already a demanding profession, and we won't allow our staff to be abused unnecessarily.

Now, let's talk about some of those yelling clients.

Yelling Client #1: The Toothless Wonder

This was the unfortunate nickname one of my mentors gave a particular client. Cruel though it sounds, it did reflect her rough appearance: mid-to-late forties, maybe early fifties, with missing teeth, tattered jeans, and a stained tank top. She owned a large white Malamute who was critically ill with immune-mediated hemolytic anemia (IMHA). In this disease, the body mistakenly destroys its own red blood cells. It can sometimes be managed, but in this dog's case, treatment wasn't going well. He had developed a severe abdominal infection, likely secondary to the immunosuppressive drugs he was receiving. Despite aggressive care, his prognosis was very poor—less than a 25% chance of survival, requiring multiple blood transfusions, surgery, and thousands of dollars in care.

When the owner came to visit, she brought her elderly mother with her. She crawled into the dog's kennel to lie beside him while I delivered the difficult news. His red blood cell count had dropped again, requiring yet another transfusion, and the infection made survival unlikely. I gently raised the subject of euthanasia, explaining that it might be the kindest option.

Her reaction was immediate and explosive. She began to sob uncontrollably, then escalated into loud, hysterical wails. Clutching the kennel bars like a prisoner, she screamed at me: *"Don't kill my dog! Don't you dare kill my dog!"* over and over, shaking the cage doors violently. Her mother tried to console her. I tried to reassure her that nothing would happen without her permission. But she was inconsolable.

Eventually, I stepped away to calm myself. There was simply no way to have a rational conversation in that moment. Ultimately, her mother signed the paperwork, giving us permission to euthanize the dog. That was the first time in my career I faced a client so distraught that I couldn't reach them. And yet, she seemed to blame me for her dog's suffering.

It was a painful reminder that clients often forget veterinarians and their staff are human too—we feel the same grief and heartbreak they do. But we do not deserve to be screamed at.

Yelling Client #2: Abby, the "Covered in Feces" Incident

Abby belonged to a rather prominent lawyer in the community—you know the type, the accident-injury attorneys you see on TV. Now, we don't change the way we care for patients based on who their owners are, but of course, when a client like this comes in, everyone is especially careful to dot i's and cross t's.

Abby needed a routine TPLO surgery (tibial plateau leveling osteotomy), one of the most common orthopedic procedures for dogs with cranial cruciate ligament injuries. The surgery went perfectly—anesthesia was smooth, the bone plate was placed exactly right, and she recovered comfortably.

She did, however, have one minor issue: post-anesthesia diarrhea. Nothing catastrophic, just soft stool. Unfortunately, Abby was also anxious and restless, so despite frequent walks, she had a couple of accidents in her kennel. Between her anxiety and her tendency to spin in circles, the mess spread more than usual. She got four baths that day alone.

When I called her owner (the wife of the lawyer) to give an update, I explained the situation and offered to keep Abby overnight. The diarrhea wasn't dangerous, but it was ongoing, and we thought she might do better at home once settled. The wife snapped on the phone: *"I am absolutely not keeping Abby in the hospital a moment longer than necessary!"*

"Fair enough," I replied. "I just want you to be aware that she's had some diarrhea and we've had to bathe her a few times." She was adamant: Abby was going home.

About an hour later, the lawyer's wife arrived. We had just bathed Abby again and gone over discharge instructions. On the way to the lobby, Abby had another small accident. We cleaned her up as best we could, but she still had a couple of tiny flecks of stool near her incision.

Five minutes later, I heard an overhead page for me, and over the intercom I could hear yelling in the background. When I got to the lobby, I wasn't prepared for the spectacle.

Picture this: a well-dressed woman in a leopard-print fur trench coat, immaculate nails, high-heeled black boots, full makeup—except the mascara, which was now running down her cheeks. She was sprawled on the lobby floor, sobbing and screaming over Abby in front of a dozen other clients:

"There's feces in the incision! My dog is covered in shit!"

My heart rate spiked—not because of Abby (who looked perfectly fine), but because of the client meltdown unfolding in my waiting room. Abby was calm and clean, save for two specks of stool no bigger than a pinhead.

Keeping my voice calm, I approached and said, "Ma'am, would you like to collect yourself? We can take Abby into a private exam room to talk about your concerns."

Everyone in the lobby was staring. Some gave her judgmental looks. She flushed bright red, finally realizing the scene she was making. As I escorted her out, three people actually applauded.

In the exam room, I asked her to show me what concerned her. She pointed to the two tiny flecks—one on Abby's e-collar and one near the incision. I wiped both away with a paper towel and scrub, all in about 15 seconds. Then I asked, "Is there anything else?"

She exploded again: "I am furious about the condition of my dog!"

I gently reminded her that we had discussed Abby's diarrhea that morning, and that she had insisted on taking her home anyway. At that, she didn't have much to say—just silence and a blank stare.

Finally, she stormed out with Abby, yelling, *"You'll be hearing from my husband!"*

Her husband, of course, was the well-known personal injury lawyer. We braced ourselves for a call. But, unsurprisingly, it never came.

Chapter 9

World "Ass" Care

So, the hospital I first joined in Milwaukee was called Animal Emergency Center (AEC). At the time I joined, it was solely owned by one of the earliest veterinarians to become board-certified in the American College of Veterinary Emergency and Critical Care (ACVECC).

When I arrived at Animal Emergency Center, there were three such board-certified individuals on staff, all of whom were my mentors and highly respected in the field. One mentor remains a good friend, though we no longer live in the same city; another, sadly, passed away after a battle with cancer; and the final one—the scariest of them all—has since become a co-author with me on a textbook that is now part of the specialty training curriculum for residents working toward the same certification I hold, DACVECC. That's something I am very proud of.

As I mentioned, I had joined this prestigious hospital to begin my three-year residency, working toward the goal of achieving board certification. To become a board-certified specialist, a licensed veterinarian must complete three years of intensive mentorship under the direction of specialists in the same field. During those three years, we spend the majority of our time working in our area of interest, building skills and knowledge, while also rotating through other specialty services such as surgery, internal medicine, anesthesia, and more. These residencies often take place at university teaching hospitals, but some large private or corporate practices, such as AEC, also have the facilities, staff, equipment, and dedicated specialists needed to train the next generation of veterinary specialists.

For practices that are not university-based, residency training must also fit within a sustainable business model so that the hospital can continue to operate. While veterinarians are rarely "in it for the money," we did choose this career as our profession, which means we go to work every day to earn a living—just like everyone else—so we can pay bills, mortgages, student loans, and car payments. This is our job, and like any job, we try to find one we love, but we also need it to support us financially.

Like any well-run business, AEC regularly revisited its mission statements and mottos to help motivate the staff and demonstrate the exceptional care we delivered to clients. At the time, the hospital was updating its motto—though I don't remember what the old one was—to the new phrase: "World Class Care." I truly believe this was a fitting motto, as AEC had been delivering world-class care since its inception. The hospital, although known by other names before my time, originally opened its doors in 1977 as a weekend and overnight emergency facility, founded by another veterinarian who would later also become board-certified in ACVECC. The specialty college of veterinary emergency and critical care didn't even exist until the 1990s, so his certification came later. As veterinary medicine advanced, the hospital expanded to a 24/7 facility in the 1980s, and from that point forward it never closed its doors.

In the early 1990s, several specialists joined the team, but emergency and critical care always remained the core of the hospital. When I joined in 2003, one of my mentors—the owner of the hospital and a founding member of ACVECC—was Rebecca Kirby. This facility was one of many things she built, and I am proud to have worked under her guidance for many years. Because emergency and critical care was always at the center of the hospital's mission, we carried forward her tradition of making AEC a premier destination for veterinary care.

Although the hospital's name has changed several times over the years, at that time we had already been recognized locally as one of Milwaukee's "best places to work," and we were the first veterinary hospital in the nation to earn certification as a Veterinary Emergency and Critical Care Society (VECCS) Certified Level I emergency facility.

So, with the adoption of our new motto, "World Class Care," the hospital hosted a large team meeting and dinner party for all employees. We went to a local restaurant with a banquet facility, where we celebrated with cake and champagne, honoring the continued efforts of our incredible team. The cake was decorated in big bold letters: "Thank you to the team of Animal Emergency Center for delivering World Class Care!"

The owner of the company cut the cake and handed a slice to everyone, myself included. When I looked down at my piece, I couldn't help but wonder if it carried a special message meant just for me. Quietly, I started to question whether my mentor liked me—or perhaps if she was trying to send me a subtle signal with this particular slice. Meanwhile, everyone else seemed to be enjoying their cake and chatting with coworkers as though nothing was unusual. But I will never forget the piece of cake I received that night.

Later, I went to my mentor and asked if she had meant something by it. We looked down at the cake together, and she burst out laughing as I finally exhaled in relief. My piece had been cut in such a way that the letters "C" and "L" from the word "CLASS" were missing, leaving my slice to read simply: "ASS."

I turned bright red, sat down, and quietly ate my piece of cake—but not before snapping a picture of it! (Figure 12)

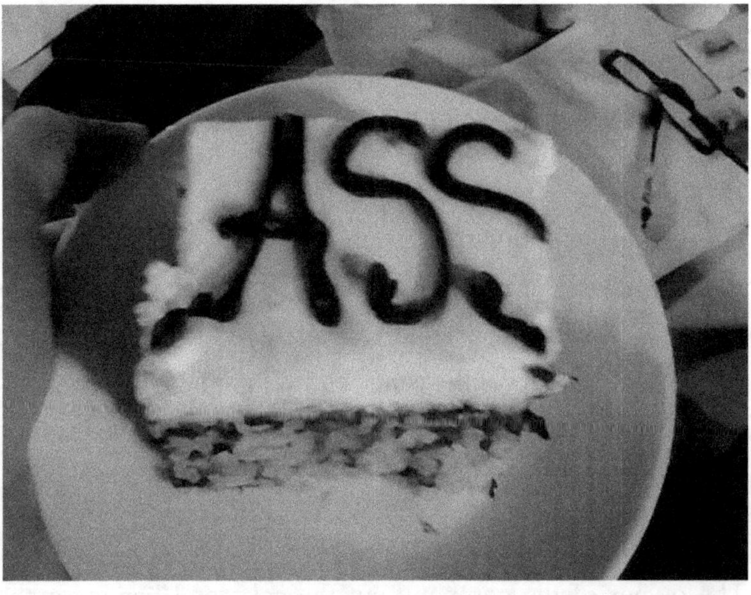

Figure 12

Section 4

Creativity in some Sticky Situations

Chapter 1

Occasionally We Use Power Tools

Most of the time, when power tools come into contact with a body—animal or human—the outcome is rarely good. Cuts, scrapes, amputations, and even death can result from accidents involving these machines. I'm sure you've all heard stories about how devastating power tool–related injuries can be. Yet, there are rare occasions when power tools, applied to a biological body in the right way, are necessary to solve a problem. And that's where this next story begins.

In veterinary medicine, the power tools we most often use are in orthopedic surgery. For example, we may need to precisely drill into bone to place a screw or attach a metal plate to stabilize a fracture. These surgical tools are specially designed: they're powered by pressurized gas, self-cooling, and engineered to minimize risk while making our work more precise and efficient. Another commonly used tool is the cast saw. Unlike a circular saw, it has an oscillating blade that moves back and forth rather than spinning. This allows it to cut through the hard, rigid material of a cast while sparing soft tissue, since skin and muscle move with the blade instead of being sliced.

Now, you might expect this story to be about a power tool gone wrong—a tragic accident or a serious injury. But it's not. This is actually a good story, a positive story about how a power tool helped us in a very unusual situation.

Several years ago, a young female pit bull named Penelope came to us after getting her leg stuck in a curled, wrought iron railing. You know the kind: thick black metal, about the width of a finger, twisted into decorative spirals for stair railings or fences. Your grandma may even have some at her house. Penelope had been roughhousing with her brother when she managed to wedge her leg through one of these coils. The owners didn't see it happen, but they heard her screams and rushed over. They found her trapped, leg twisted awkwardly in the railing. In her panic, she thrashed so violently she made the entrapment worse—and even broke several teeth while biting at the metal in desperation.

Eventually, she calmed enough for the owners to approach. They tried wiggling her leg free but it wouldn't budge. Desperate, they grabbed a hacksaw. Thankfully, they didn't try to cut her out directly. Instead, they sawed through the railing to detach the section trapping her leg. With the bar still wrapped tightly around her carpus (wrist), they carried her—leg and iron bar still attached—to the hospital.

When Penelope arrived (Figure 1), the bar was clamped firmly around her leg, leaving her unable to move it at all. There was already a small skin wound—whether from the struggle, the railing, or her own chewing was unclear—but the bigger concern was what happened next. Within minutes, her leg began to swell rapidly, almost enveloping the bar. If blood supply were cut off completely, amputation could have been inevitable. We had to move quickly.

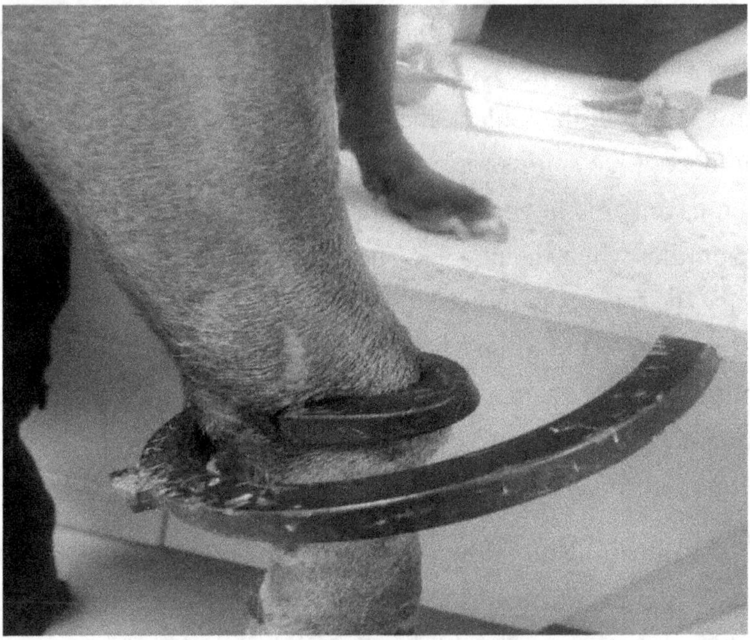

Figure 1

We placed an IV catheter to give sedation and pain relief. Even so, it was clear the discomfort was too severe for her to tolerate manipulation. She needed to be fully anesthetized. Within minutes we had induced anesthesia, intubated her, and connected her to monitoring equipment.

Now under anesthesia, we tried every conservative trick: twisting, pulling, lubricating, even attempting to bend the bar. Nothing worked. The leg was locked in place.

That left us with one option: power tools. At first, we considered the cast saw, but its oscillating blade wasn't nearly strong enough to cut through three-quarters of an inch of solid wrought iron. A Dremel-style rotary tool was also inadequate; the attachments we had couldn't handle the job. The only solution was a heavy-duty rotary metal-cutting saw. We didn't normally have one in our medical toolkit, but our building manager kept one for maintenance. Without it, our next step would have been calling the fire department. Thankfully, he brought the saw to us, and we prepared for a delicate operation of a very different kind.

Whenever we perform a risky procedure, we remember the principle of "first, do no harm." But in this case, there was no way to completely shield Penelope's leg. The swelling had ballooned around the bar, making it impossible to fully protect her skin from the blade. Adding to the challenge, rotary saws generate significant heat, which could easily cause burns. Every move had to be deliberate and precise.

With Penelope anesthetized and her leg as protected as possible, we started the cut. Sparks flew as the blade bit into the metal (Figure 2). We worked slowly, pausing frequently to cool the bar and blade with water. This not only reduced the risk of burns but also gave us time to check that her leg remained stable and safe. We wore protective eyewear, fixed her leg in place, and draped a wet towel over her head to shield her from flying sparks.

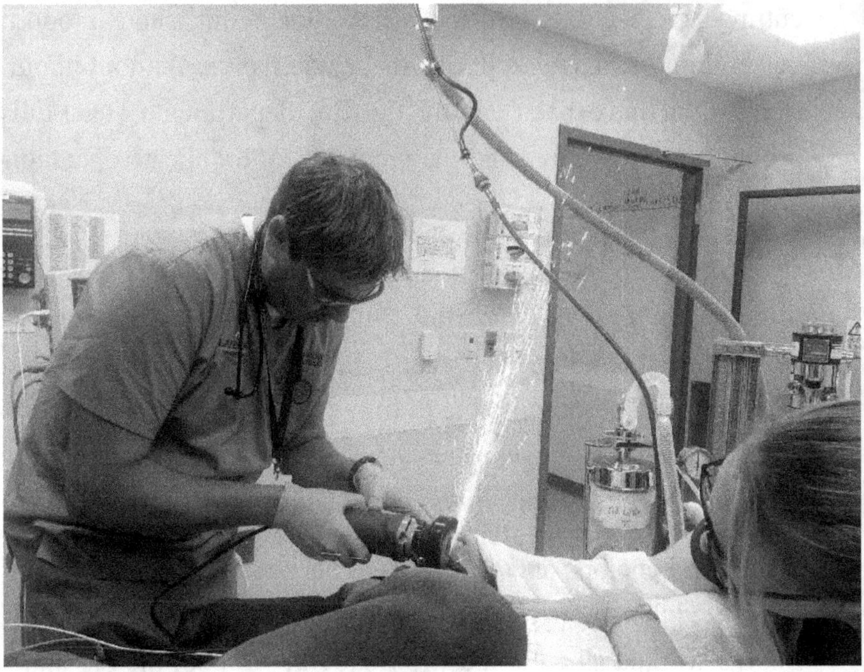

Figure 2

But one more danger loomed: oxygen. Pets under anesthesia are given supplemental oxygen, either flowing freely near their mouth if sedated or delivered directly to their lungs via an endotracheal tube if intubated, as Penelope was. With sparks flying, any free oxygen in the room could have ignited, causing an explosion. Fortunately, because she was intubated, the oxygen was contained within the circuit rather than escaping into the air. Still, it was a constant concern as we worked.

Bit by bit, we cut deeper into the bar. For most of the length, we managed to slip padding between the metal and her skin. But at the deepest point, where her swollen leg fully wrapped around the bar, padding wasn't possible. I had no choice but to make a small incision in her skin to allow access for the final cut. I felt guilty about it, but the alternative was far worse: losing her leg. Once the cut was complete, we used pliers to bend the bar apart. At last—success! The bar released, and Penelope's leg was free.

A cheer erupted from the team. But the work wasn't done. Penelope had several small wounds on her leg and face, as well as the minor incision I had made. We cleaned the injuries, administered local anesthetic (lidocaine), sutured the small cut, and started her on antibiotics and pain medication. She also received a supportive bandage. Later, she would need dental surgery to address the teeth she had fractured in her panic.

In the end, Penelope made a full recovery. With time, proper care, and plenty of love, she healed completely. Today she's a normal, happy dog—living proof that sometimes, the right tool in the right hands can save a life.

Chapter 2

Some Super Sticky Stuff!

Veterinary medicine is full of sticky stuff, and every once in a while, patients come into the hospital because they have gotten themselves into some of it. Sometimes, it is really sticky stuff. This is the tale of three patients who found themselves in very sticky situations.

The first two were slithery species: snakes. Snakes are amazing creatures, and people tend to be quite polarized in their feelings about them. They either love snakes or they hate them. One of the first things most people learn when handling a snake is that they are not slimy. Touch one, and you quickly realize they are scaly. Which means that if they get into something sticky, it clings to them and does not just slide off. If you are the owner of a snake, you need to be careful about what those non-slippery serpents might find themselves slithering into.

The stories of these sticky snakes are fairly simple: they slithered by something too sticky, it got all over them, and they wound up in trouble.

The first snake was a corn snake who lived up to his reputation as an escape artist. He kept slipping out of his terrarium. No matter how many times his owner put him back, the snake would slither up the side, find the spot where the black plastic grate covering his enclosure popped loose, and escape again. Frustrated, the owner tried a series of DIY fixes to secure the mesh covering to the glass-sided tank. The final solution? Duct tape.

We have all used duct tape, and it is wonderfully versatile, but it is not meant for securing snakes in their cages. This time, duct tape tricked the serpent into a sticky predicament. You can see in the attached photo (Figure 3) how the snake first arrived at our hospital.

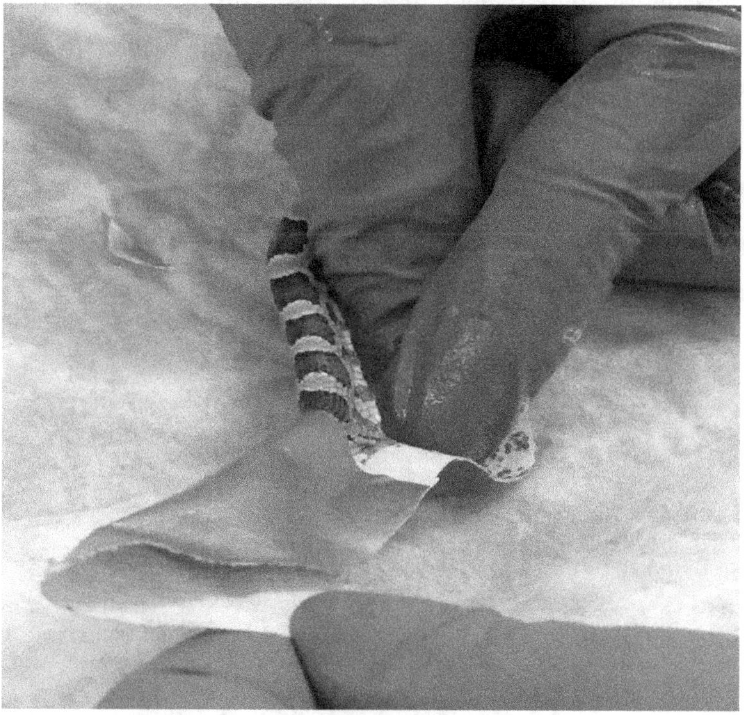

Figure 3

When he came in, he was tightly wrapped and badly contorted. His face was stuck inside the tape, and about two to three inches of his head and body were bound in the mess. He had already twisted himself further into it, pulling the tape over his nares and close to his mouth. Had it gone a little further, he might not have been able to breathe. You can imagine how quickly it could have become life-threatening, like having your nostrils and mouth taped shut. At the moment, he was still breathing fine, but he was anxious and struggling. With a lot of patience, teamwork, and, admittedly, a bit of swearing, we managed to save him before the tape did real harm.

Surprisingly, he remained cooperative throughout and did not require sedation, which made the process easier. It still took multiple hands, plenty of patience, some soap, and a gentle solvent to peel him free without damaging his scales. Slowly but surely, we extricated him from his duct tape prison. The second picture (Figure 4) shows him lying on a paper towel, finally free.

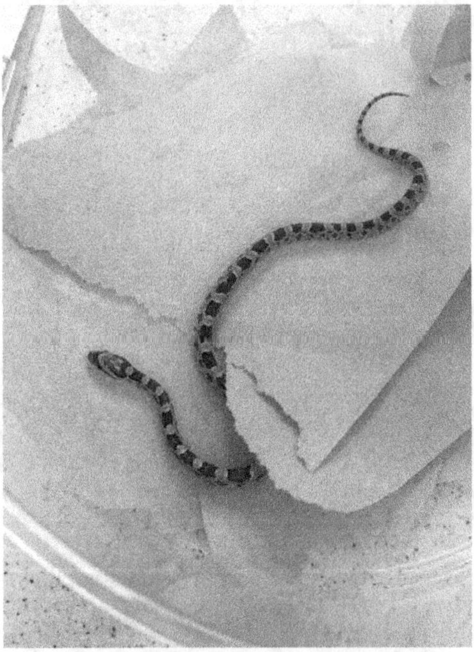

Figure 4

The second snake, curious as ever, ended up in a similar mess. Like the corn snake, he also managed to escape his enclosure.

The timing could not have been worse for his owners. They were also dealing with a mouse infestation in their home. I have been in that situation myself, so no judgment. We joked at the hospital that perhaps the snake had escaped in hopes of helping with the problem, since many snakes naturally eat mice. I imagine he had seen a few rodents scurrying around and thought it looked like an easy snack.

Unfortunately, the owners did not see it that way. They set out mouse traps, including sticky traps, to catch the rodents. If you have never used them, these are pieces of adhesive-coated cardboard or small boxes with bait. A mouse walks through, gets stuck, and is unable to free itself. The snake, after escaping, found one of these traps and became the unintended victim. The more he struggled, the more hopelessly he was caught.

The photo (Figure 5) shows this unfortunate snake, a ball python, wrapped in adhesive from the trap. Ball pythons are one of the most popular snake species to keep as pets. They are generally friendly, do not bite, and often bond closely with their owners.

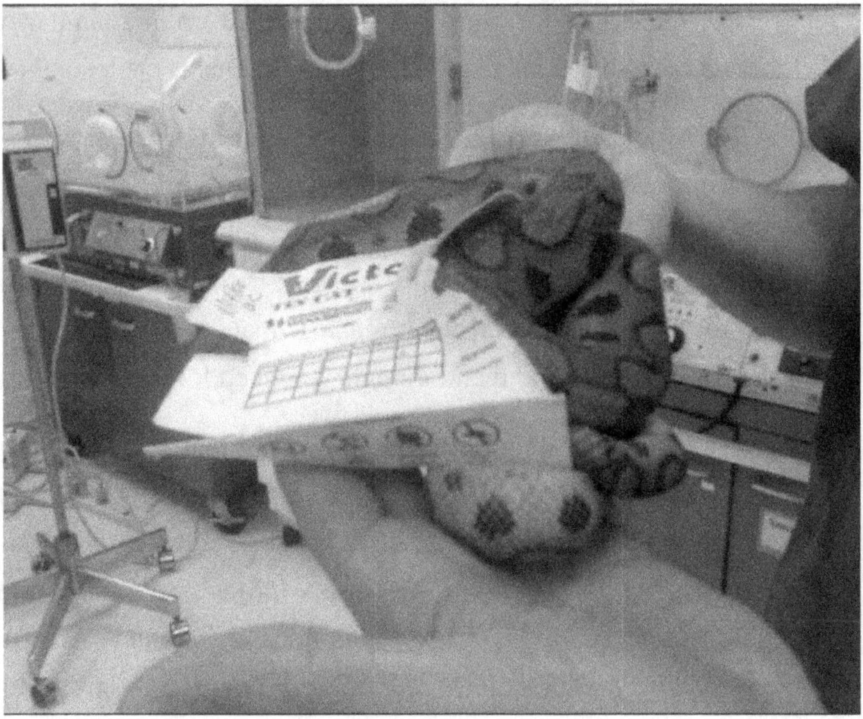

Figure 5

This snake did require a little bit of sedation, because he was so tense and wrapped up in the trap. After the sedation kicked in, it took quite a long time and significant perseverance to peel this mouse trap off the snake, or vice versa. With more soap and gentle solvent, we were able to free him without causing any injury. Once he recovered from the sedation, he was able to go home without any lasting issues.

The third tale in this trio of sticky situations was a one-year-old male hound mix, about 50 pounds in size. Like so many other dogs, this one ate something he should not have eaten. Just like some kids in early elementary school, he developed a taste for something sticky—glue. Why? I can't really say, for the same reason I don't understand why some kids eat glue. I guess it just tastes good to some animals. As I often remind people, dogs lick their own butts, so how bad can glue really taste to them? I don't have children, but I imagine having a dog or cat must be a lot like having a two-year-old. They get into anything and everything, and sometimes that includes glue. One of the most common types we see ingested in the hospital is Gorilla Glue. This particular type is important because when it hits the stomach, it hardens into a rock.

We took radiographs, or x-rays, of this dog's abdomen shortly after he arrived. If you're not familiar with canine radiographs, a typical lateral view, where the dog is lying on its side, will show the head to the left and the tail to the right. In a view where the dog is lying on its back, the head is usually at the top and the tail at the bottom. For this dog, I circled the stomach in the images, which was very dilated and filled with a mixed-density mass of "stuff" (Figures 6 and 7).

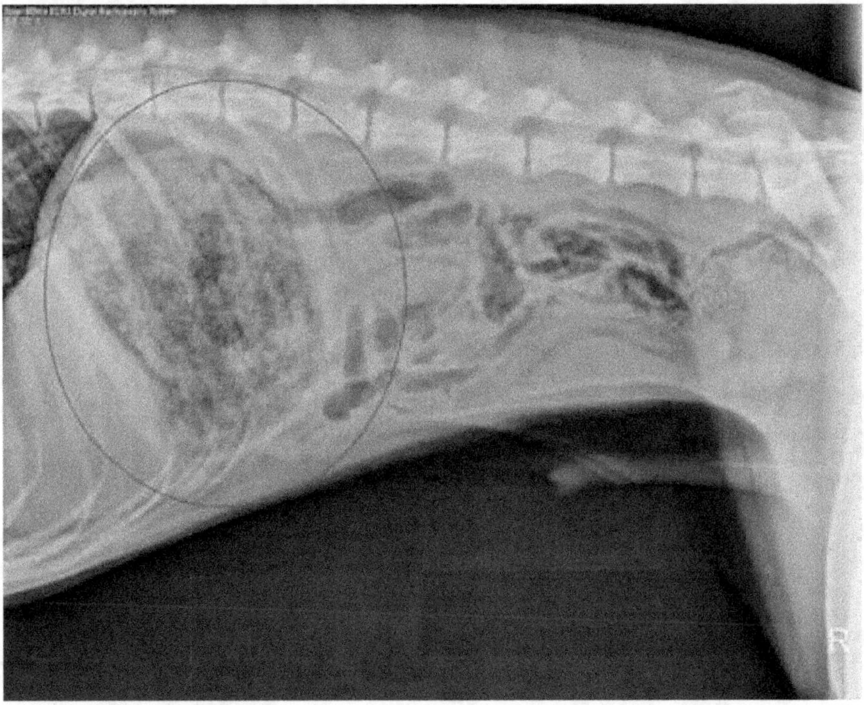

Figure 6

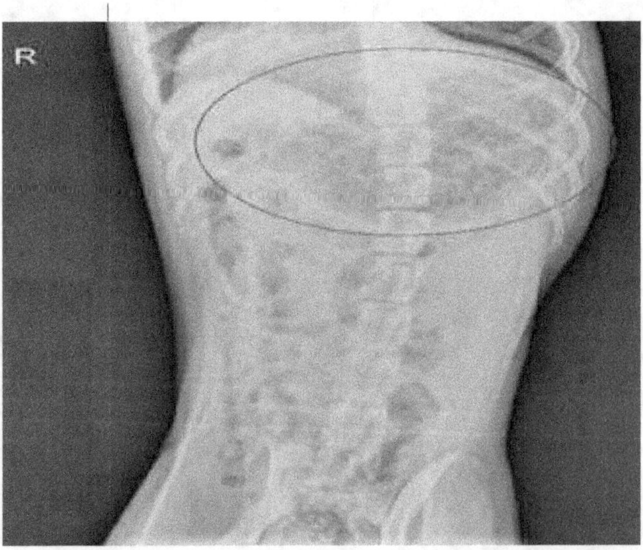

Figure 7

The problem with radiographs is that a lot of things in the stomach look the same. Food, socks, dirt, and even glue can appear identical, since they all share the same density as tissue or fluid mixed with gas. In this case, we suspected the material was glue but couldn't be 100 percent certain. The good news was that the glue itself is not particularly toxic, though it can cause vomiting and abdominal pain.

This dog wasn't vomiting, painful, or uncomfortable, so we decided to monitor him for a short time. We did call an animal poison control center to confirm there wasn't anything toxic in this particular glue. They also advised against inducing vomiting, since Gorilla Glue hardens into a large, firm mass that is often too big for a dog to bring back up.

When we rechecked x-rays the next day, the mass hadn't changed in size. The dog had only been given water and no food during that period, so if the material had been food, it should have been digested and the stomach smaller. Because it hadn't changed, we were concerned that the hardened glue was causing an obstruction, and we strongly recommended surgery.

The owners agreed, and surgery proceeded fairly routinely. Once we opened the abdominal cavity, we could feel a large, firm mass inside the stomach. We made a sizable incision into the stomach to remove the foreign object, and as expected, we found a hardened mass encompassing most of the stomach's interior. You can see in the photo (Figure 8) that the mass was about twice the size of an average fist.

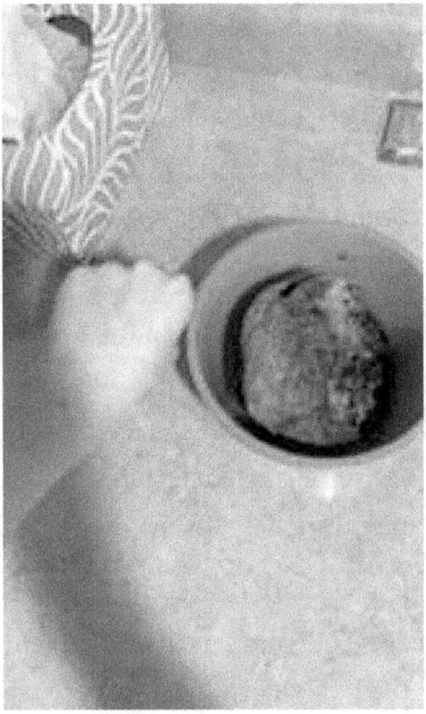

Figure 8

Fortunately, this dog had an uneventful recovery and was discharged the next day. As always, we cautioned the owners to keep whatever "tasty" objects their dog found far out of reach. Dogs rarely learn their lesson after one of these episodes, even if it means going through surgery.

Chapter 3

Other "Stick-y" situations

Dogs in their modern lives tend to get a little bored. We ask them to lay around all day while we are at work, and not as many people as should are willing to take them for a much-needed walk after a long day at the office. Some modern options for exercising our restless companions include sending them to doggy day-care, or, as many people prefer, taking them to the dog park. Either way, the hope is that they get the exercise they need. Dog parks certainly have many advantages, but they do come with disadvantages as well. Feel free to ask your veterinary professionals about those drawbacks, I am sure they would be happy to share. Still, dog parks are a great way to socialize your dog while providing both mental and physical activity, though they can also present hazards and risks of injury.

What do dogs do at the dog park? They run. They run and run and run, just like children after a long day cooped up in a classroom, needing to burn off energy. They romp and play, chase each other, and have a great time. But sometimes, running at top speed and being a silly dog can lead to serious trouble. Let me tell you about three more "stick-y" situations that dogs have gotten themselves into at the dog park.

If you have never been to one, picture the average dog park. They can be found in both urban and rural settings, though many are located in suburbia. Typically, they are fenced-off areas of land that often include natural woods, and sometimes even a stream. Most of the time, they are quite nice, enjoyable for both pets and their owners.

When I lived in Wisconsin, the average dog park there tended to be a little larger than those in big cities. In places like Chicago or New York City, dog parks are generally smaller, but still often contain at least a couple of trees, which becomes important a little later.

Many dog parks also include plenty of open spaces for running. Those open fields, however, can occasionally cause problems. I specifically recall two greyhounds that visited an open-field park and, according to their owners, collided in a full-speed, T-bone-style crash. The collision did not end well for either dog. The first suffered a broken neck, while the second fractured his scapula, or shoulder blade. Both belonged to the same family and required a tremendous amount of care to recover from their injuries. Situations like this remind us why it may actually be beneficial that many dog parks also contain wooded areas, as trees and brush can break up the space and prevent dogs from colliding at top speed.

For most dogs and their owners, though, it is not as enjoyable to have only an open field. That is why many parks include trails for people to walk while their dogs explore. In hotter regions, trees and bushes also provide much-needed shade, as well as added aesthetics. These forested areas divide the park into several regions, give dogs interesting obstacles to run around, hiding places for squirrels and wildlife, and spots to mark with urine. Unfortunately, those same trees and bushes can also present dangers, as dogs may trip, crash into them, or, in the worst cases, impale themselves on branches or sticks.

I have personally seen dogs run headfirst into trees and bushes, sometimes tripping or colliding when they were not paying attention. In the most severe cases, dogs can impale parts of their body on sticks. The three dogs in the stories that follow each impaled their face in some manner, with a large stick lodged into one of their facial orifices.

It seems that Labradors are particularly prone to this type of injury. Perhaps it is a breed disposition, or maybe it is simply because Labradors are so common. They are, after all, one of the most popular breeds. Bred as working dogs, they need plenty of exercise, and while many are intelligent and benefit from the mental stimulation parks provide, Labrador owners will agree that sometimes they are also just a little bit clumsy. Do not get me wrong, Labradors are among the best family pets you can have. I owned one myself, and he was a loyal companion who loved to run, but even he had his share of "not so smart" moments.

The first story took place on Valentine's Day. While most people remember that holiday for spending time with loved ones and sharing flowers and chocolate—though remember, chocolate is toxic to dogs—I remember it for removing foreign objects from several canine faces.

The first patient was a Labrador who had been running through brush at the dog park when his owner noticed he suddenly started sneezing violently. The dog pawed at his nose, and soon the owner saw a small amount of blood coming from one nostril. Concerned, they brought him to our hospital immediately. Our physical exam confirmed the findings, and after talking with the owner, we suspected there was a foreign object lodged up his nose.

As you might expect, when a dog's face is painful or uncomfortable, he is not willing to let you take a close look at his nose or mouth while awake. For that reason, we often have to heavily sedate or anesthetize these patients to properly examine the affected area. The canine nose is long and cavernous, and it is extremely difficult to see far inside. We often start with an otoscope, the same device doctors use to look into ears, but it only allows us to see the first few centimeters of the nasal cavity. For a deeper look, more advanced tools are needed.

This patient was anesthetized so we could safely examine him. Using the otoscope, we did not see much, so we escalated to a rigid metal rhinoscope, several inches long with a small camera and grasping tool at the tip. Even under anesthesia, some dogs reflexively move their head during this procedure, but once our patient was stable, we carefully examined the nasal cavity. We quickly found what we were expecting: the tip of a large stick.

It was challenging to grasp, but once we managed to secure it, we began extracting the foreign body. To our surprise, it just kept coming. The stick was much longer than we imagined. In the end, we pulled out a four-and-a-half-inch stick lodged deep inside this poor dog's nose.

He recovered quickly from anesthesia and was undoubtedly more comfortable, though his nose remained a bit bloody for a few days due to ruptured blood vessels. I am certain he was relieved to be rid of that massive stick. Unfortunately, we did not get a picture of this particular case, so you will have to take my word for it. The stick, however, was very similar in size to the ones shown in the next two stories. Be advised before looking ahead, those images are a little graphic.

Dog number two was a similar situation, a yellow Labrador running full speed around the dog park, sometimes within the owner's view and sometimes not. When she came back from her run, she was squinting her eye and would not let the owner look at it. They knew something was wrong and brought her right away to the hospital.

When we first had a look at her, the eye was so painful that she would not allow us to examine it either. Her eye was clamped shut, as tightly as she could possibly close it. We could not even get the slightest glimpse of what was going on. We had to give this Labrador pain medications and eventually heavily sedate her, just to get an idea of what was happening. We were worried about the worst, since a penetrating injury to the eye often means the eye might need to be removed if it is ruptured.

Once she was sedated, we were able to get a closer look and saw a stick in her eye socket. We weren't even sure if her eye itself was injured, as all we could see was the stick. We knew we were going to have to work carefully and cautiously to avoid any further damage. We did not know how large the stick was, how far it had penetrated into the socket, or if the eyeball itself was compromised. We had to proceed with the utmost care.

Because the tip of the stick was nearly half an inch in diameter, it was hard to imagine there would not be significant damage. We were worried she might be blind in that eye if it were permanently injured. In the first picture (Figure 9), all that could be seen was the broken end of the stick, with no visible eyeball at all. The eye might even have to be surgically removed, and in the worst-case scenario, there is a direct connection from the back of the eye to the brain. It was at least possible she had sustained a brain injury.

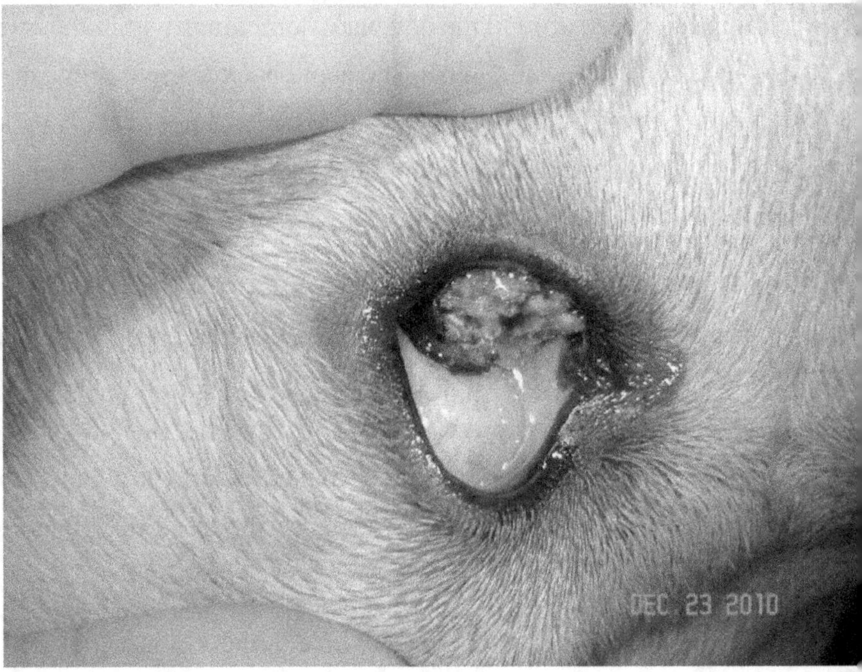

Figure 9

We worked slowly and judiciously, doing our best to protect the eyeball as much as possible. I even used a tip from an ophthalmologist friend of mine: we cut a piece from a Styrofoam cup and used it as a guard between the stick and the remainder of the eye. Under sedation, we could see the eyeball itself was pushed to one side, with what appeared to be only minimal injury.

With cautious precision, steady progress, a lot of patience, and maybe a little luck, we grasped the stick firmly, protected the eye, and slowly removed the stick from the socket. To remove it, we not only had to protect the eyeball, but also the surrounding tissues: the muscles that control eye movement, the optic nerve, and the glands, all of which could suffer significant harm. As we maneuvered the stick aside and identified the eyeball, we wedged that Styrofoam guard between the stick and the eye so we could continue safely. Slowly but surely, we made progress, and once we got about halfway out, the stick started to slide more easily until it finally came free (see Figure 10).

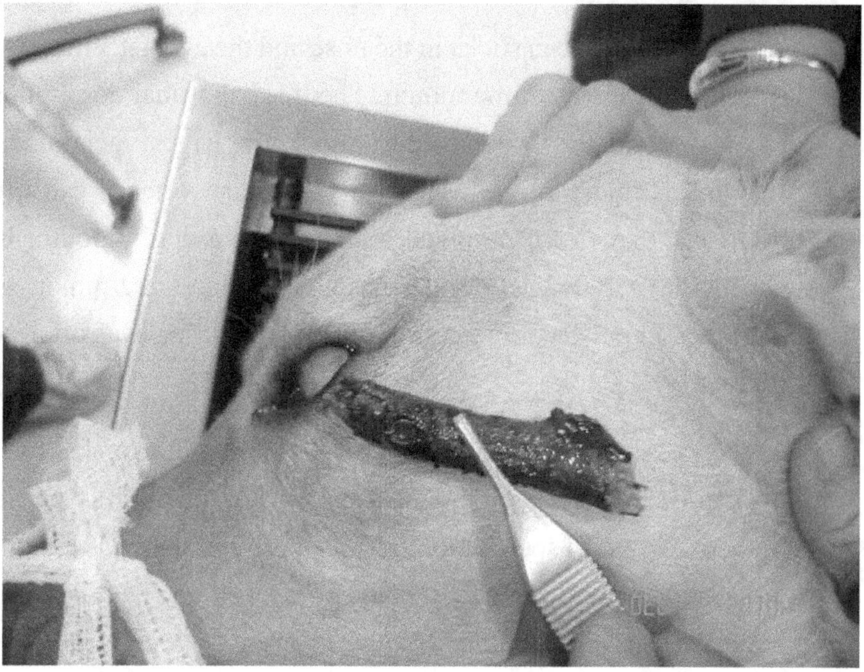

Figure 10

The stick ended up being nearly two and a half inches long. It was hard to believe how large it was and that it hadn't penetrated back into her brain.

We ran a final series of tests to check the eye itself. Miraculously, there was only minor injury to the tissues surrounding the socket, and the eyeball was intact. I still cannot believe that entire stick had been lodged in her orbit without causing major damage. In the end, she was a very lucky Labrador who did not need her eye surgically removed.

I am confident this poor pooch had a terrible eye ache and headache for a few days, so we prescribed pain medications and antibiotics to prevent infection. She recovered just fine.

Now, having seen sticks in the nose and the eye, let's move to the last orifice of the face: the mouth. The third and final dog in this set of "stick-y situations" managed to impale the largest facial opening. This type of injury is one we actually see fairly often. I can't recall how many times I've removed a stick from a dog's mouth, but it happens on a somewhat regular basis. Most cases are minor, like a stick wedged between the teeth. This one, however, was on a whole different level.

Don't ask me why Labradors run full speed into sticks, but they do. You'd think they would be smarter than that. This particular Labrador ran at full speed, mouth wide open, and stabbed herself with a large stick under the tongue. Feel free to view the next picture, but be warned, it is quite graphic (Figure 11). The stick pierced the tissue beneath her tongue and traveled about three additional inches, making this stick the largest of the three I've removed from a dog's face. Its total length was five to six inches, with about half embedded under the tongue.

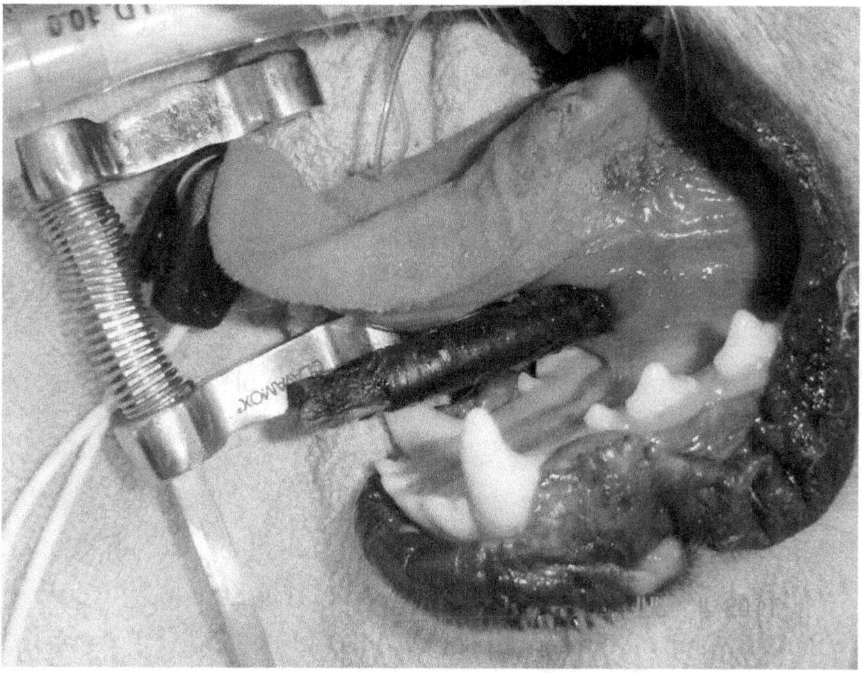

Figure 11

Some sticks are simple to remove, they slide right out. Others are far more challenging, especially if they have thorns or small branches, which can splinter off inside tissue and cause more harm.

This case was more difficult than the nose or the eye. After sedating the Labrador, we tried a little gentle traction, as with the previous two cases, but this stick would not budge. The first two sticks came out slowly with careful maneuvering, but this one resisted. I had to put on my "oral surgeon" cap and make a few incisions under the tongue to enlarge the puncture wound so the stick could be safely removed.

If you are not aware, the oral cavity has a very rich blood supply. When the tongue, mouth, or gums are poked or cut, they can bleed quite a bit. While it can look alarming, this blood supply is actually beneficial because the mouth harbors loads of bacteria. With the extra circulation, oral wounds are more resistant to infection and tend to heal quickly.

After making precise incisions and applying steady, gentle maneuvering, we finally removed the stick in one piece, thank goodness. We flushed the wound thoroughly, inspected for any leftover thorns or fragments, controlled the bleeding, and sutured the wound closed.

All three of these dogs were extremely fortunate despite their injuries. Each went home with pain medications and antibiotics, and each healed quickly. With some skill and a little luck, we were able to get them all out of their "stick-y" situations.

Chapter 4

Missy and the Medication Mix-up

We get a lot of interesting presenting complaints (reasons why animals need to go to the vet), in the veterinary ER which makes every day feel unique. Sometimes an animal gets into something they shouldn't, and sometimes owners give them something they shouldn't. What always strikes me as curious, particularly with the availability of "Dr. Google or Google AI" these days and the vast amount of information on the internet, is why people will give their dog something like ibuprofen, or worse yet Tylenol (acetaminophen), and then look it up afterward to see if it was safe.

Why doesn't it occur to them to check before giving it? And if they thought it was okay beforehand, then why look it up afterward? Why not just check in the first place, or better yet, call a veterinary clinic and ask? We are always happy to share when home remedies are appropriate and let you know if something is safe for your pet. Preventing toxic ingestions before they happen is so much easier than treating the consequences. In these cases, prevention truly is better than cure, and a little foresight goes a long way.

Regardless, it seems that more often than not, someone calls after they have already given their pet something unsafe. That is where we come in. My point here is just a word to the wise, a small reminder to help prevent these situations.

Missy's owners were a little different. They had simply made a mistake. So, let's start with Missy's story. She was a middle-aged to older, white, fluffy mixed-breed dog. Her owners noticed she had been squinting her eye for a couple of days and had already taken her to their primary care veterinarian. There, some redness and squinting, called blepharospasm, was noted. She was diagnosed with a simple scratch to the cornea, the clear part of the eye, and prescribed a topical ointment to treat it.

For those who haven't had a dog with a corneal ulcer or scratch, it sounds much worse than it usually is (most of the time). Although it can be uncomfortable for the dog for a short time, for the veterinarian it is a straightforward problem to diagnose, and for the owners, usually simple to treat. Most of these injuries heal fairly quickly.

The diagnosis of a corneal ulcer or scratch involves applying a green stain called fluorescein to the surface of the eye. The stain sticks to the ulcer and highlights it bright green, so it can often be seen with the naked eye, or with the help of a blue light. This is shown in Figure 12, where the large green spot in the middle of the eye is a corneal ulcer.

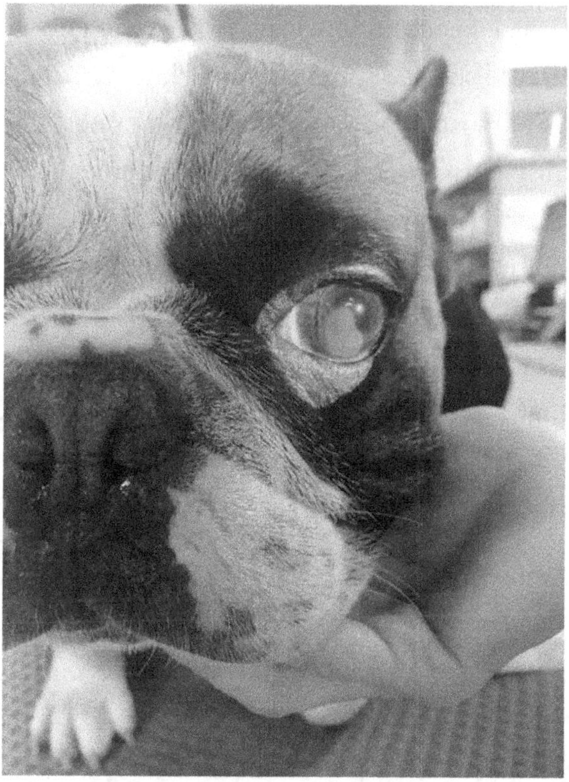

Figure 12

Most corneal ulcers are caused by a minor scrape or a small particle stuck to the eye, and they are usually a simple fix. Medication alleviates the discomfort, prevents infection, and allows the ulcer to heal. Most resolve within a few days. Some dogs, however, are predisposed to corneal ulcers. Short-nosed breeds, called brachycephalic dogs, such as Pugs and Boston terriers, can be more prone due to decreased tear production or because their eyes protrude slightly from their flat faces, a condition called exophthalmos. Their eyes tend to dry out more easily, making them vulnerable to ulcers.

Missy had been slowly losing her vision for years, and her owners believed she had simply bumped into a chair at home, causing the injury. For most dogs, partial vision loss is not a big deal and they can live fairly normal lives. Even dogs that are completely blind can navigate their environment well and live happily. The challenge comes when furniture is moved, which can throw off their bearings and lead to accidents. Missy's owners were in the middle of some home renovations and had moved furniture around, so it made sense she might have bumped into something and injured her eye. No big deal, right? Accidents happen. But this accident was about to get much worse.

As I mentioned, Missy's veterinarian diagnosed a corneal ulcer and prescribed ointment to be applied several times a day. For the first two days, things were going fine. Then, during one attempt to apply the ointment, the mix-up occurred.

A little background helps explain what happened. The owners had been repairing some wooden items at home, including furniture and a picture frame. For this, they had been using super glue.

Most people are familiar with super glue. It usually comes in a small tube, not unlike a miniature tube of toothpaste. You squeeze the bottom, and a little glue comes out. Eye ointments come in very similar-looking tubes. Unfortunately, Missy's owners mixed up the tubes.

You can probably see where this is going, but it gets a little worse than you might expect. If you have ever tried to put eye medication in a dog's eye, you know it is not easy. Dogs usually resist, especially if the eye is sore. They squirm, move their head, and clamp their eye shut. Applying ointment often becomes a two-person job. But half the time, only one of Missy's owners was available, and it was always a struggle.

Because of this, they would squeeze out a large amount of ointment around the eye, hoping that enough would get inside to be effective. No criticism to the owners here, this is just how tricky it can be. In fact, they had already needed refills because so much medication had been wasted during application. Veterinarians understand this and often provide refills for that reason.

The same struggle occurred during the mix-up. Missy was thrashing her head, and the owner managed to get a big glob of ointment in and around her eye, on the fur and eyelids as well.

Afterward, Missy walked away squinting, just as she normally did after treatments. The owner grabbed a wet towel to clean her face, but when they called her back and tried to wipe her fur, they noticed the ointment was unusually firm, sticking stubbornly to her hair. It didn't wipe off like it normally would.

That is when they looked at the tube, and I'm sure their hearts sank. They had mixed up the eye ointment and the super glue. They had just applied super glue directly into Missy's eye.

Needless to say, they rushed to package Missy up, called us in a panic, and came flying into the clinic, understandably hysterical.

Even in the ER, we sometimes encounter things we have never seen before. For all of us on duty that day, this was one of those times. Honestly, we were worried about the potential outcome. Certainly, super glue in a dog's eye does not sound good. We were glad Missy was on her way so we could help, but we had no idea what to expect when she arrived.

We were also glad her owners called ahead, which gave us a few minutes to consult textbooks. Unfortunately, none of them offered much guidance. There was no published information we could find about treating an eye contaminated with super glue. So, we waited until Missy arrived, prepared to assess the situation firsthand.

It was every bit as bad as it sounded. Missy was uncomfortable but surprisingly tolerant, yet the glue was everywhere. It coated her fur, sealed her eyelids shut, and seemed to be on her eye as well. In the first picture (Figures 13 and 14), her eyelid is glued closed. The second photo, taken later during the exam, shows the eyelids opened. Because the glue had dried semi-opaque, we could not actually see the eyeball itself, which made the assessment even more challenging.

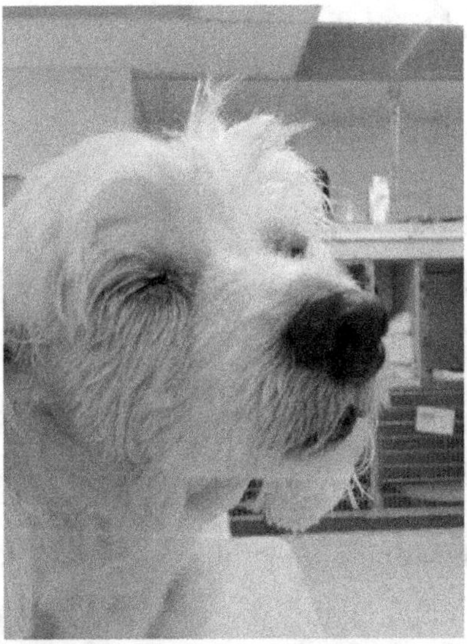

Figure 13

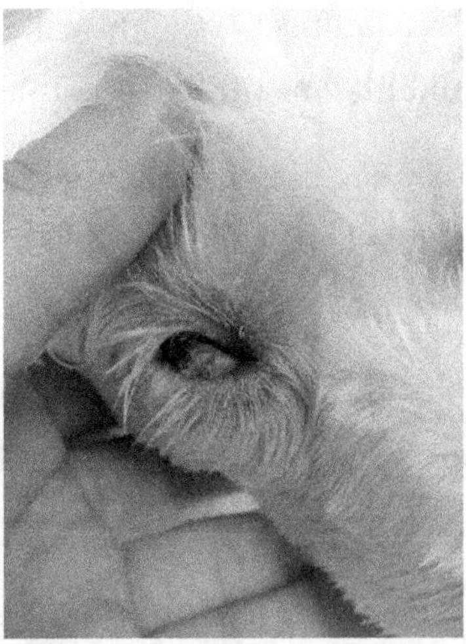

Figure 14

We happened to be particularly lucky in our clinic, as we also had a veterinary ophthalmologist we could call for help in situations like this. We knew we had some tough work ahead of us, but we weren't sure how to proceed. We administered pain medication to Missy, which also sedated her a little, and she allowed us to use a solvent and scissors to remove the glue from around her eye. We clipped some of the fur to open her eyelids just enough to attempt visualizing her eyeball.

That was when we called the ophthalmologist, not knowing what to expect. Would we have to remove her eye? Was this causing irreparable damage to her cornea, potentially rendering her permanently blind? How painful was it? Was there anything we could do?

On the phone, one of our doctors frantically described the situation while trying to remain calm. After listening, the ophthalmologist simply replied, "Yeah, she'll be fine."

What a sweet sigh of relief that was for us, Missy, and her owners. As it turns out, during the development of ophthalmologic surgical techniques, there were times when surgeons struggled with how to surgically close the eye after it had been opened. In those days, superglue-type solutions were sometimes applied directly to eyes to help with closure. Advances in technology have since allowed us to use microscopic sutures instead, but the fact remained—glue had been used before in ophthalmology.

Of course, we had to keep in mind that not all types of superglue are safe. Some are harmful, some less so, and we were fortunate that the glue Missy's owners used was one of the less harmful types. All we needed to do was clean the glue off her eyelids and fur, and her eye would be OK.

That may seem hard to believe. But if you've ever gotten sticky glue on your fingers, you know that after a few days it eventually just comes off. This happens because skin cells naturally shed and replace themselves, and the glue loses its grip. The same process occurs with the cornea—the cells replace themselves just like skin cells.

Now, this doesn't mean it's safe to put glue in the eye. As I mentioned, some glues can be very damaging, and we had to confirm that this particular type did not contain dangerous solvents or chemicals.

Some glues are safe enough for medical use. In fact, we sometimes use skin glue to close small wounds. But that doesn't mean you should ever try fixing problems on your pet with glue—please do not do this. Every glue is different, and some are much worse than others.

For Missy, all we had to do was place an e-collar to prevent further injury, administer longer-acting pain medications, and continue the antibiotic ointment she had already been prescribed. Admittedly, applying it was a little trickier with glue still in the way.

What a surprise and relief it was for all of us. We were able to assure her owners that Missy would be fine, though her healing would take time and she would be uncomfortable for a while. A few days later, her owner called to report that Missy was already doing better, though some glue remained in her eye. Ten days later, at a recheck with her veterinarian, the glue had nearly all fallen away, and the original ulcer had healed.

Sometimes there is a little good luck even in a bad situation, and we were all happy to hear that Missy came through the medication mix-up just fine.

Chapter 5

You and Me Doing Surgery in The Dark

Our hospital was going through major renovations a few years ago, and at the same time we had a number of very intense spring storms. These storms frequently knocked out the power, and over the course of three to four months we lost electricity nearly ten times that spring. It was simply bad timing—while we were dealing with repeated outages, we were also updating major electrical components in the hospital, including a new backup generator. Unfortunately, there was a delay in its installation, and our old generator was no longer up to the task. The outages happened so often that we had to revise our hospital's power-outage protocol.

This is a story of veterinary innovation.

During this series of outages, we had to get creative. I've been through so many power failures in my career that they no longer bother me, but for less experienced staff members, it was unnerving. What may surprise many people is just how much medicine—and even surgery—you can still perform without electricity. Many of our instruments run on pressurized air or batteries, anesthesia can be delivered by injections or pressurized gas, and several devices have battery backups. So we could still do quite a lot without power. Of course, we couldn't run advanced imaging like CT scans, mechanical ventilation, or MRIs, but there was still plenty we could accomplish.

That said, batteries only last so long, and monitors are among the first things to fail. We could still place IV catheters and administer medications since most in-hospital medical care is delivered by hand. We could even keep fluids running, but instead of infusion pumps, we had to rely on gravity drips from fluid bags. That required close monitoring, carefully counting drips per second or per minute to maintain accurate rates.

Even major soft-tissue surgeries could continue, since they're performed entirely by hand. Orthopedic surgeries, however, were more challenging. We often rely on electrical tools like cautery, and without them we had to adjust. We also couldn't use anesthesia ventilators or run most bloodwork. Manual ventilation was possible but exhausting for staff, and only the simplest blood tests could be performed on battery-powered equipment. In short, losing power didn't throw us back to the dark ages, but it did feel a lot like being in a 1960s military hospital.

Because of my experience, I wasn't particularly shaken when outages occurred, but newer staff members were understandably nervous. The biggest problem of all, however, was lighting. Nearly all hospital lighting runs on electricity, and we don't have a good substitute for it. Emergency lights provide just enough to move safely through the building, but not nearly enough for doctors and nurses to work effectively. Good lighting is critical to nearly everything we do.

Normally, we were prepared for short outages thanks to our backup generator. It was actually a solid system in design. Unlike many generators that run on gasoline, ours ran on natural gas hard-wired into the building, giving us a constant fuel source without relying on electricity. It also had a self-regulating mechanism, so within ten seconds of a power loss it would automatically switch on. The generator didn't power the entire hospital, but it supplied designated red outlets, emergency lighting, and other essentials. That gave us enough to function, even if equipment requiring heavy power, like the CT scanner, laundry, or most computers, stayed offline.

But as we learned that spring, nothing is infallible, and even backup systems can fail.

During the renovations and those storms, our aging generator was put to the test—and it failed several times. Usually, when the power went out, I would start counting to ten, confident that by the end everything would roar back to life. But three or four times that spring, I counted to ten, then twenty, and then a full minute, before realizing there was a problem with our generator.

Eventually, we learned it was a minor mechanical issue. It was repaired once, then again, and again, before engineers finally resolved it. At the time, though, it hardly felt minor. We knew the generator was old and already scheduled for replacement, but the new one hadn't yet been installed, so we were stuck managing outages with an unreliable system.

Most of the time, the outages occurred during quieter evening hours, which was a small mercy. But several patients were under anesthesia when the power failed, and that was always a serious concern.

As a critical care doctor, it's my job to remain calm in moments like this. Still, when the lights go out mid-surgery and silence closes in, keeping everyone steady is no small task.

One evening, near the end of an orthopedic procedure, the power failed again. We paused and began our usual count to ten. Nothing. Frustration swept through the room as the generator failed yet again. But the ER team didn't hesitate.

In today's world, everyone carries a cell phone, and within seconds the room filled with beams of light as staff rushed in, flashlights blazing. It was just enough illumination to let the surgeon finish the operation without skipping more than a beat or two.

I'll never forget that moment. Standing back, watching my team surround the table, their faces glowing under the pale glow of phone flashlights, I felt proud and grateful. I even snapped a picture—one more reminder of how innovation, teamwork, and a little quick thinking can turn a crisis into a success (Figure 15).

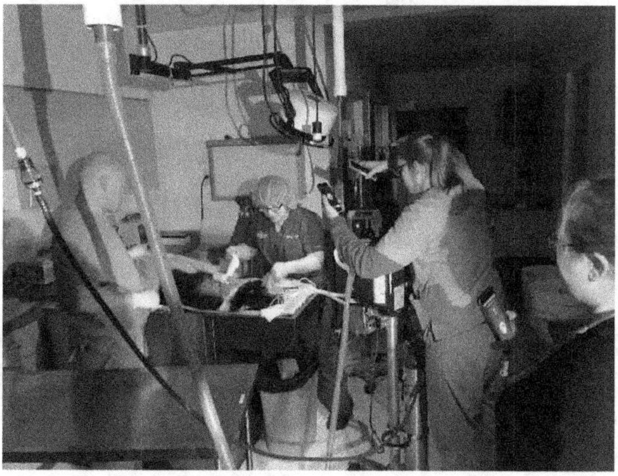

Figure 15

Chapter 6

A unique method of body care

Not too recently, I hospitalized an older dog who, as it turned out, had a very serious problem. Through several blood tests, we diagnosed him with a disease called immune-mediated hemolytic anemia, or IMHA. This is a very serious condition in which the body's immune system mistakenly recognizes its own red blood cells as foreign invaders. The immune system then attacks and destroys those cells. Patients with IMHA quickly become very sick and severely anemic, which often means they need to be hospitalized, placed on injectable medications to suppress the immune system, and in many cases, given blood transfusions.

Most of the time, we start medications to suppress the immune system so the body will stop breaking down its red blood cells, but these medications take time to work. The challenge with this disease often comes down to the cost of ongoing treatment. Hospitalization, medications, and especially transfusions, while waiting for the drugs to take effect, can become very expensive. In the meantime, while waiting for the medications to work or while trying to find the right combination, these patients suffer the consequences of their red blood cells being destroyed. This can lead to several complications: 1) blood clots, which is why they are often placed on blood thinners, 2) jaundice from the breakdown of blood cells, which makes pets very ill, and 3) the most common and most dangerous, anemia. A dangerously low red blood cell count can result in shock or even death.

If a patient destroys enough of their red blood cells, transfusions become necessary, and with large dogs, this can get expensive very quickly since they may need multiple transfusions. Dogs and cats have blood types similar to humans, and blood banking techniques are also similar. We can collect and store blood for them, but it is costly and time-consuming. As a result, repeated transfusions quickly become unaffordable for many pet owners.

The good news is that the prognosis for this disease has improved dramatically. When I was in veterinary school, we were taught that the survival rate was about 50%. That meant half of the animals diagnosed either died or were euthanized, which was devastating. Today, thanks to advances in medical care, survival rates have climbed to 80% or more. That is a huge improvement.

This brings me back to the patient in question: Buddy, a very cute, middle-aged pit bull. If you haven't figured it out by now, pit bulls are one of my favorite breeds. They're incredibly friendly dogs. Buddy had been diagnosed with IMHA and was brought to our hospital. After running the appropriate workup, we confirmed that he was destroying his own red blood cells. When I explained the diagnosis to his owner, she was devastated. She kept asking, "Why? Why Buddy?" These are some of the hardest questions to answer, because most of the time there is no clear reason. Sometimes IMHA is triggered by tick-borne disease, cancer, toxins, or another underlying issue, but often it's simply the immune system malfunctioning without explanation.

Our discussion continued. Buddy needed to be hospitalized on intravenous fluids and medications to try to get the disease under control. We also discussed the possibility of transfusions. Ultimately, the owner decided she could afford the initial testing and one transfusion, but no more. The difficulty was that there's no way to predict how many transfusions a patient will need. Some require none, others one, and some many. We have to monitor red blood cell counts and clinical signs very closely. If we see abnormal heart or respiratory rates, or other symptoms of severe anemia, another transfusion may be required.

On Buddy's first day, we were able to hold off on a transfusion. By the second day, however, his red blood cell count dropped from 20% to 12% (with normal being around 40%), and his heart rate was elevated.

Buddy's owner came to visit, and I met her in the room to discuss his condition. She was happy to see him, though clearly disappointed with the news. She wanted to continue his care despite knowing there was a real risk Buddy might pass away or need to be euthanized. She asked many questions about euthanasia and aftercare, and this is where things took an unexpected turn.

Some of her questions were typical: "What is the process like? How fast is the injection? Does it hurt?" But then she shifted focus toward body care, which is something we usually discuss only after an owner decides on euthanasia.

"What happens after they're euthanized?" she asked. I explained that most people choose cremation, though some choose home burial if permitted by local regulations.

“Do people ever take them home?” she asked.

“Sometimes,” I said, “but usually when they’ve planned for home euthanasia followed by burial. You just have to check with your municipality, since burial isn’t allowed everywhere.”

She nodded and then said, “Well, I’m not thinking about burial. I’m thinking about an alternative.”

I paused, wondering what she meant. Alternative options do exist, but they’re uncommon. I’ve had a handful of clients ask about taxidermy, and though it comes up occasionally, very few actually go through with it. To each their own, I always say. In teaching hospitals, we sometimes ask for permission to perform a necropsy or use the pet for training so students can learn procedures on cadavers, which is an invaluable experience for young veterinarians. I’ve even had four clients inquire about cloning, though that’s rare and extremely expensive. Still, none of these seemed to match what she had in mind.

Her idea was something I had never encountered before.

She explained, “I’m an archaeologist, and I have a particular interest in archaeological sites that contain both human and animal remains. They tell fascinating stories about ancient diets and about our bond with animals.”

“Interesting,” I said. “Go on.”

“Well, what I was wondering,” she continued, “is if I could skeletonize my dog if he gets euthanized.”

I froze. Then paused again. Then again.

Finally, I admitted, "This is a question I've never even considered, and I don't have an immediate answer."

Most of us have seen animal skeletons in museums, and I've always found them fascinating, both personally and professionally. They offer valuable insight and are routinely used in veterinary education. But I had never once been asked about skeletonizing a personal pet.

I knew I needed to respond carefully, so the question didn't linger uncomfortably in the air. I explained, "There's a lot to consider if we were to go down that path." My brain immediately started racing through the practical and legal implications.

"You mentioned you're an archaeologist. Do you know of facilities that could perform this?" I asked.

She nodded. "Yes, there's one here in the city. I could probably get access, and I'm sure I could get grad students to help with, you know, de-fleshing the body."

The thought of graduate students de-fleshing their supervisor's pet—or any pet—was unsettling, but she spoke about it calmly, from a purely scientific perspective.

"OK," I said, "we can consider it, but there will likely be regulations to review. One concern is that euthanized animals contain chemicals from the injection, essentially poison, which would have to be disposed of safely through incineration. We may also need to consider alternative euthanasia methods to ensure safety."

Digging deep into my memory, I recalled the skeletonization process: first, the bulk of the tissue is removed manually, then beetles clean away the remaining tendons, and finally the bones are bleached. I added, "I'm not sure how the euthanasia solution would affect the beetles used in the process. It's possible the tissue could be toxic to them."

We discussed the idea further but ultimately ended with me saying, "Let's hope it doesn't come to that. We don't need to make this decision right now."

Fortunately, Buddy needed just one more transfusion that night, and after that, he stopped breaking down red blood cells. He went home with his owner the next day, and the last update I received was that he was doing well.

I suppose I was lucky we never had to go down the path of figuring out how to skeletonize a dog, though I immediately shared the story with my colleagues. We all felt a little sympathy for the grad student who might have been asked to take on such a task—an experience they were unlikely to forget.

Section 5
Exotic Species and Other Select Stories

Chapter 1

Creative Solutions For A Burrito

(Or When I Learned How To Fork A Pig)

We are one of the few companion animal hospitals in the region that will see "exotic" pets, particularly on an emergency basis. Most of our time is spent treating dogs and cats, however, being willing to see exotic animals means we are prepared to help nearly any species when an emergency occurs. There are a few limitations to this though, since we are only able to see animals that we have the proper facilities to restrain. For example, we cannot properly restrain a horse or a tiger in our hospital, but there are many other species we can help, such as goats, pigs, birds, small mammals, lizards, and more.

To give a little background on veterinary education for exotic species, most veterinarians during school, or sometime shortly after, usually end up choosing a small animal focus, such as dogs and cats, or a large animal focus, such as horses and cows. Some working in rural settings end up treating both, and a few veterinarians are fortunate enough to work primarily with exotic species. For most of us, seeing these unusual animals is a rare privilege and a challenge, which makes it a bit exciting when something non traditional comes into the clinic.

To be willing to examine and treat exotic species, each veterinarian has to be comfortable with tackling situations they may have never faced before. Creativity and flexibility are often required, since many things that apply well to one species do not apply at all to another.

And so, with that background, here begins the story of Burrito. In late 2019, we received a call from an owner with a pet pig named Burrito. The owner had called several other veterinary clinics before contacting us, none of which were willing to see him. As happens often with owners of exotic species, they struggled to find a facility willing to treat their pet for an emergency, especially on a weekend. But Burrito's problem could not wait several days, or even several hours, as his life could quickly be in jeopardy.

The problem was that Burrito had gotten into rat poison on the farm where he lived. When the owner called, the front desk staff, unsure whether we would see this particular species, paged me over the intercom to ask if it was all right to bring him in. I reluctantly agreed, since I had only seen one or two pigs in my career, and I knew what kind of challenges we might face.

When Burrito arrived, he was bright, alert, and responsive, or "BAR" as we say. He was a medium-sized pig, estimated at about 60 pounds, mostly black with a white collar of hair around his neck and a bright pink belly and limbs (Figure 1). His physical exam, as much as you can determine from a pig, was fairly normal. This was definitely a good start considering the challenges that lay ahead.

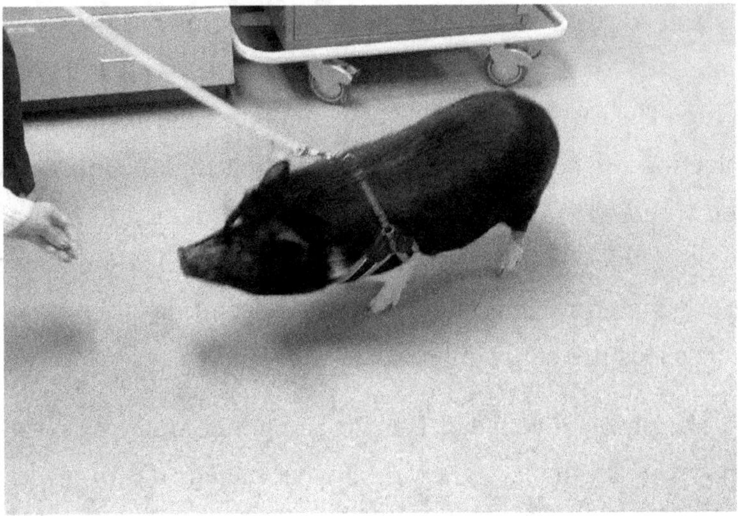

Figure 1

You must understand a little about pigs before we continue, since I am sure most readers have not had much hands-on experience with them. Pigs are smart and friendly, but they are also extremely determined animals. Maybe stubborn is a better word, since determined underestimates how challenging they can be. Trying to make a pig do something it does not want to do is no small task. If the pig is uncooperative, you need luck on your side, and you definitely need ear protection. When pigs resist, they squeal, and the squeal of a pig is not cute or endearing, but closer to a scream. A pig's squeal can reach 115 decibels, which is louder than a jet engine and potentially damaging to your ears if sustained.

Now, back to Burrito's problem, the rat poison ingestion. When any patient comes in for rat poison exposure, the first step is to determine what type was ingested. There are dozens of different rodenticides, each working through different mechanisms. Most people do not realize that these poisons are not immediately fatal.

Their toxic effects take time, sometimes days, before symptoms begin. This is why it is critical to see the patient as soon as possible. We do not want to wait for symptoms to appear, because by that point the patient's life may already be at risk, and treatment becomes far more complicated and costly.

Burrito had ingested an anticoagulant rodenticide. Any animal that eats this type of poison, including rats, pigs, dogs, or humans, develops an inability to form normal blood clots, but this takes several days to appear. An inability to clot may not sound serious at first. After all, many people are prescribed anticoagulants like Plavix® or Warfarin to prevent clots, which can be beneficial in controlled doses. But too much of a good thing can be fatal. These rodenticides were designed to kill, and they work the same way in nearly all mammals. In the case of anticoagulant rat poison, if a large enough dose is ingested, the animal cannot clot blood at all and will eventually begin bleeding internally.

Why does this happen? All mammals constantly rupture tiny blood vessels throughout the body. Normally, clotting factors, proteins made by the liver and always present in the bloodstream, step in to seal those holes. Once the vessel is repaired, the clot is broken down through fibrinolysis. But when anticoagulant rodenticide is ingested, the body can no longer make new clotting factors. Eventually, the supply runs out, and countless tiny ruptures in the capillaries begin bleeding unchecked. Once enough of these occur, the animal bleeds to death internally. The process usually takes days, and because the bleeding is internal, there are no outward signs. At first, the animal may just appear weak and pale, with an elevated heart rate. But as more blood is lost, shock sets in, and death follows.

The good news was that Burrito was not in immediate danger, since he had only just ingested the poison. Still, we had to act quickly to prevent bleeding from starting. The first step in any toxic exposure is to determine whether enough of the substance was ingested to be harmful. To do this, we calculate the dose by dividing the estimated amount of toxin by the animal's body weight, giving us a milligram per kilogram (mg/kg) measurement. That requires two things, an accurate body weight and an idea of how much was consumed.

Getting a body weight on a pig, however, is easier said than done. We tried everything to get Burrito onto the scale, tempting him with food, tugging gently on a leash, even pushing with our knees. Burrito was having none of it. This was when the squealing began, and it was so loud we had to use earplugs just to continue working. Pigs are not only stubborn, but strong, and despite several attempts, we could not get Burrito onto the scale. In the end, Burrito won the battle, and we had to estimate his weight instead. After calculating, we determined that the amount of poison ingested was indeed high enough to be potentially lethal, which meant further action was urgently needed.The next step with exposure to any toxin is decontamination. With an ingested toxin, this means making an animal vomit to decrease the contents in the stomach, followed by the oral administration of activated charcoal to prevent further absorption of the toxin. With dogs and cats, it is fairly simple to induce emesis (vomiting). We give them an injection of medication, and within just a few minutes vomiting occurs, emptying most of the contents of the stomach. Inducing vomiting is more challenging with many species, and unfortunately, it is nearly impossible with pigs. Pigs do have the ability to vomit, but there are no simple injections we can give to cause it reliably. It is also very challenging to find a vein in which to administer the medication, which makes it even more complex. (By the way, did you know it is nearly impossible for some species to vomit, such as rabbits and horses?)

Here we were, in this challenging situation: we could not weigh Burrito and we could not make him vomit, so our only option for decontamination was to feed him activated charcoal to bind to the toxin in his stomach and hope that it would be sufficient to prevent internal bleeding.

This presented our next challenge with Burrito: how do you make a pig eat charcoal? We thought it would be easy at first. With most of our patients, we can either add the charcoal to a little bit of food and they will eat it, or we have to syringe it into their mouth manually. It is often a messy process, with charcoal getting all over us, the patient, and the towels we use to contain the mess. There was no way Burrito was going to allow us to restrain him so we could syringe the charcoal into his mouth, we knew he would fight and squeal the entire time. So, our only choice was to try mixing the charcoal with canned chicken and dog food in the hope he would eat it on his own. We tried, but Burrito had no interest in eating the "slop" we made for him. He was too worked up by that point, anxious and probably a little mad. Our options were becoming very limited, but we all wanted to help Burrito avoid a toxin-related crisis.

There is a third option for administering activated charcoal, through a feeding tube, but this requires either a very cooperative patient (which Burrito was not) or brief general anesthesia. At that time, I was not going to get into the complexities of anesthetizing a pig, and I will not now, except to say that putting Burrito under anesthesia was likely too dangerous and unnecessary. We just needed a creative solution.

This is when I learned how to “fork a pig.” Please read that carefully, fork. I am sure forking a pig is not what you are thinking. As it turns out, one of our veterinary technicians on duty that evening also owned a pot-bellied pig and knew a trick to help pigs relax, forking them. She took Burrito into a quiet room, away from the hustle and bustle of the clinic, and let him explore until he was comfortable. Eventually, he laid down. This is probably where you imagine she put on some Barry White and lit candles to help him relax, LOL. Nope, neither of those things happened.

To calm Burrito, the technician brought a fork into the room and began gently poking and scratching him with it, hence the term “forking a pig.” He loved it. It was like a relaxing little piggy massage. He calmed down, relaxed in his new environment, and finally, we were able to coax him into eating the activated charcoal to prevent absorption of the toxin. Check out the picture (Figure 2)! Yes, that is a fork in her hand, scratching Burrito’s belly.

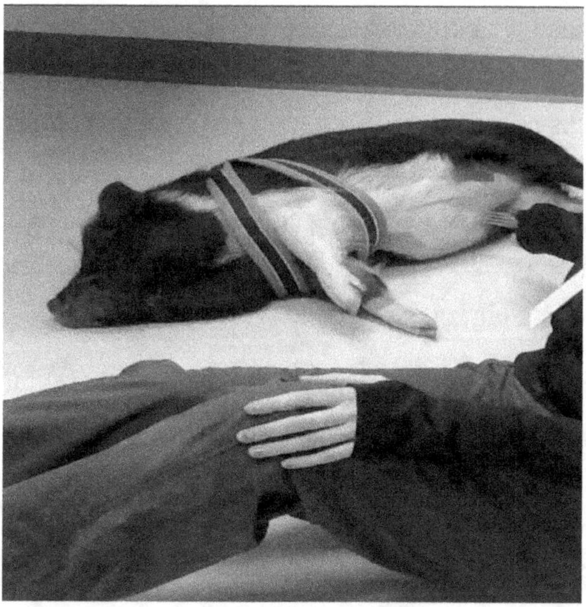

Figure 2

After Burrito finished his charcoal meal, we sent him home. His owners were so thankful that we were able to help that night. However, Burrito still needed to be monitored closely at home. With most patients who ingest anticoagulant rat poison, post-exposure monitoring is always recommended. With dogs and cats, we typically measure blood clotting times at two different points: at ingestion, and again two to three days later. This ensures there is no risk of bleeding and allows us to identify a problem before it occurs. If clotting parameters are normal, no further treatment is needed, but if they are prolonged, the antidote must be started. With successful decontamination, it is actually rare that an antidote is required. A veterinary study showed that only 8% of animals need it when treated within six to eight hours of ingestion.

Because we could not make Burrito vomit, we were not certain the charcoal alone would be enough. We also knew Burrito would never let us poke him with a needle to check his blood clotting time, for three reasons: 1) he was stubborn, 2) it is difficult to draw blood from a pig compared to other species, and 3) normal clotting times for pigs are not as well established as they are for dogs or cats. Oh, such a troublesome pig.

Since we could not reliably monitor Burrito's clotting, we turned to the antidote. Very few toxic substances have one, but anticoagulant rodenticides do. The antidote is phytonadione, also known as Vitamin K1. Typically, we only give Vitamin K1 if clotting times are abnormal, but in Burrito's case, we did not have much of a choice, since we were not completely confident the charcoal decontamination worked.

We sent Burrito and his owner home with a prescription for Vitamin K1, which they would have to administer every day for 30 days. This particular toxin is very long lasting, so the full course was necessary. The owners were more than happy to comply, knowing it could save Burrito's life.

That night, although we had faced some pretty big obstacles, we all felt good knowing we had helped another family and another pet. And Burrito had enjoyed a nice, relaxing forking session too.

Chapter 2

Freddie Mercury in Infamy

I've had the opportunity to work with many species over the years, and even a few celebrities during my days in Los Angeles. At the hospital where I worked, the celebrities who came in while I was there included Eric La Salle (Dr. Benton from *ER*), one of the Wayans brothers, Courteney Cox, and my favorite by far, Bob Barker. I will save the story of Bob Barker for another book, as it deserves its own telling, but for your viewing pleasure, I've included a picture of myself with him and my parents (Figure 3).

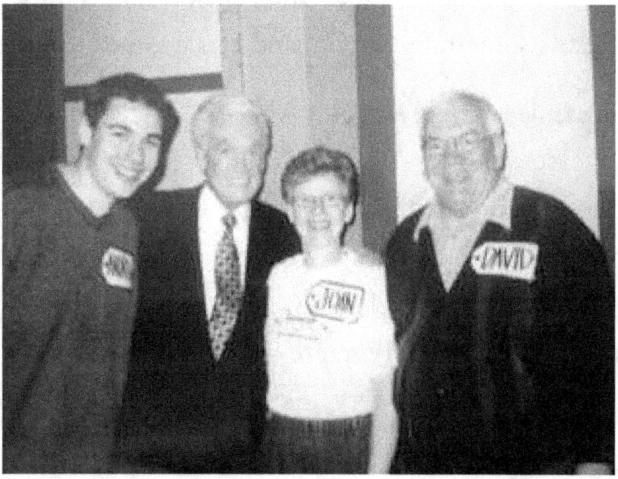

Figure 3

Although this story is named after a famous singer, the Freddie Mercury in this story became known for a very different reason. It is also a story of veterinary ingenuity, and one that eventually landed me on national television. That is how I came to meet and treat the infamous Freddie Mercury.

Of course, this Freddie was not the legendary frontman of Queen, but a tortoise, more specifically an African spur-thighed tortoise, also called a Sulcata tortoise. These tortoises are named for the hard, pointed projections along their legs.

One day, Freddie came to our hospital because he was "not feeling well." That vague description is one of the trickiest parts of veterinary medicine, because it does not tell us much. Vomiting and diarrhea point toward the gastrointestinal system. Excessive drinking and urinating suggest the endocrine or urinary system. Limping tells us to look at the musculoskeletal system. But "not doing well" could be almost anything. In veterinary medicine we sometimes use the shorthand ADR, which stands for "ain't doin' right." That simply means there's something wrong, and it is up to us to figure out what.

At the time, we had a doctor who specialized in exotics, so he led Freddie's case, but I was able to work closely alongside him. Freddie had not been eating well, and as part of the diagnostic workup we performed radiographs. The images revealed several rocks and screws sitting in Freddie's stomach. Those objects were almost certainly the problem, and unfortunately, there is only one way to get them out of a tortoise's stomach: surgery. You can actually see the x-rays of Freddie with the foreign objects inside (Figure 4).

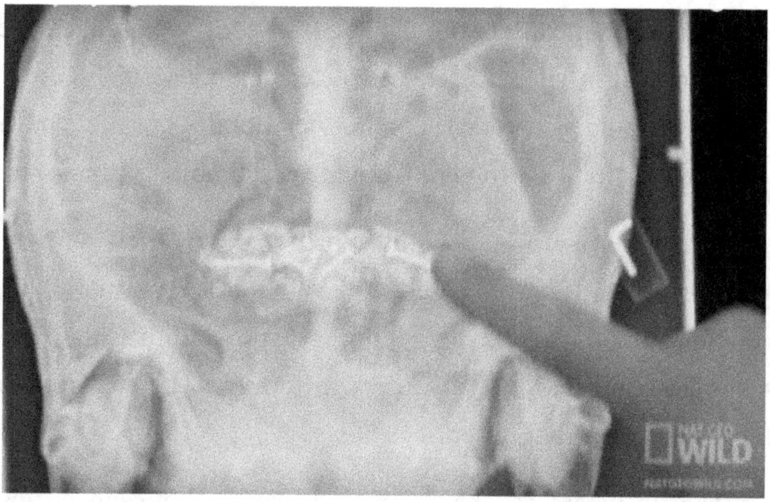

Figure 4

Surgery in dogs and cats is straightforward. We cut through skin, the layer of fat and tissue beneath, and then the body wall to enter the abdomen. A scalpel does the trick. With a tortoise, the situation is much more complicated. To reach the abdomen, we have to go through the plastron, the hard shell covering the tortoise's underside. That shell is bone-hard, which means getting inside requires a bone saw. The saw is powered by compressed air and demands a steady hand, since you must be careful not to overheat the tool or the tortoise's plastron.

I was fortunate to be working under the guidance of our exotics specialist, who performed the surgery while I assisted. Even so, anesthesia in tortoises is its own challenge, so it was another factor we had to carefully manage.

Before surgery, we had to collect bloodwork to confirm the diagnosis and to ensure Freddie could handle anesthesia. Drawing blood from a tortoise is not easy, but Freddie was cooperative. The complication came afterward: a large bruise, or hematoma, developed at the collection site. This raised a serious concern. Freddie might have a clotting disorder, such as hemophilia, or he could have developed a clotting problem from the metal objects in his stomach.

That put us in a difficult position. We knew surgery was necessary, but if Freddie could not clot his blood normally, he might bleed to death during the procedure. The problem was that very little is known about clotting disorders in tortoises, because they are so rarely studied or diagnosed.

This is where my background in emergency and critical care medicine came into play. Coagulation disorders have always been one of my favorite areas of study. I've published and lectured extensively on the subject, so I was eager to apply that knowledge.

In tortoises, however, we had to lean on what we call comparative medicine: taking what we know about other species and applying those principles where data is lacking. In dogs and cats, specialized blood tests can identify clotting problems, but no such validated tests exist for tortoises or other reptiles. Even if we ran a test, we would have no baseline values to compare against. Diagnosing the cause of Freddie's bruise was essentially impossible, so instead we had to focus on how to treat it.

In most species, if a patient may bleed excessively during surgery, we prepare with transfusions. The problem was that no one had ever reported a blood transfusion in an African spur-thighed tortoise, nor did we know whether tortoises even have blood types. If they did, an incompatible transfusion could make Freddie worse, or even kill him.

Still, we knew transfusion was likely the only way to safely proceed with surgery. That left us with one very important question: where could we find tortoise blood?

At that time, Milwaukee had a remarkable place called Hoffer's, part pet store and part exotic zoo. They carried everything from food and toys to elaborate housing and costumes for unusual pets. More importantly, the owner kept several large Sulcata tortoises on-site. In the summer, visitors could even feed and interact with them outdoors.

We contacted the owner and explained the situation. Without hesitation, he volunteered three of his tortoises. In exchange for a free health exam, we could collect blood from them for Freddie's transfusion.

The donor tortoises were surprisingly cooperative, and we collected enough blood for cross-matching. That step was critical, because while we did not know if tortoises had blood types, we could at least check compatibility between the donors and Freddie. To our relief, the blood was a match.

With that reassurance, we proceeded. Freddie received the transfusion before surgery and tolerated it beautifully. No reactions, no complications. With his clotting ability supported, we moved ahead with anesthesia and surgery. Cutting through the plastron was slow, steady work, and removing the screws and rocks was painstaking, but Freddie handled everything remarkably well.

Afterward, he recovered steadily in the hospital. We monitored him closely for infection and made sure his incision, including the plastron cut, was healing. Like bone, it takes weeks for a plastron to knit back together. Slowly but surely, Freddie regained his appetite and strength. Eventually, he was well enough to return home with his family.

The challenges were many, but in the end, we had performed what at the time was one of the very first documented blood transfusions in a tortoise. Since then, other reports have emerged in the veterinary literature, but when we searched at that time, there was nothing. Freddie's case required collaboration, creativity, and a little boldness, and I remain proud of the role my team played in his recovery.

And yes, Freddie's story became something of a minor celebrity moment. The case was featured, dramatized of course, on *National Geographic – Wild.* I had the chance to work with them a few times in my career, and it was always exciting. If you are curious, you can still find Freddie's episode on the show *My Dog Ate What?* or watch the clip on YouTube:

https://www.youtube.com/watch?v=Pn1pUcWY4wE&t=63s

Chapter 3

Travis, stop biting my face

Well, I don't have a picture of the actual patient (Travis) for which this chapter is named, but I do have a picture of one of my favorite doctors, Dr. F (as we'll call him), who helped manage this case. In the photo, he's restraining one of the few goats we ever saw at the clinic (Figure 5). That particular goat came in lethargic and anemic, and we later discovered he was loaded with intestinal parasites, but that's a story for another day. You can see the excitement on my technician's face, she's the same person who taught me how to fork a pig, she got excited whenever a farm animal came through our doors.

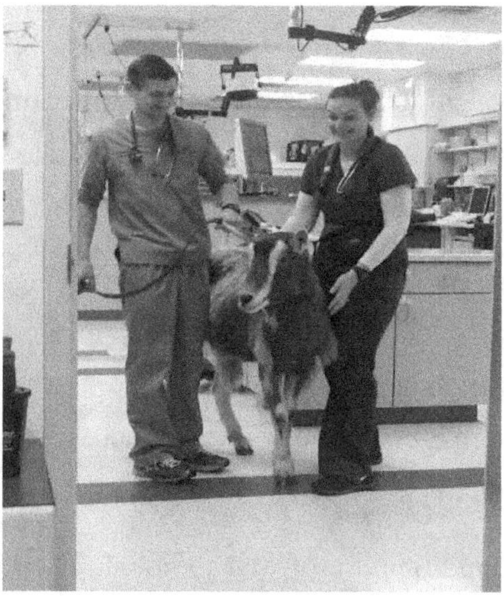

Figure 5

Travis was a two-year-old macaw. Now, macaws up close can be very intimidating animals. They have incredible strength in both their claws and jaws, and can cause serious injury if not handled correctly. Their beaks exert enough force to crack hard nuts, like Brazil nuts, and could just as easily break a finger. And if they can break a finger, they can certainly do damage to a face. That detail becomes important later.

Travis came in for what seemed like a minor problem. He had gotten his claw stuck in a piece of metal on his cage at home, causing a small injury to his toe, but it kept bleeding and needed medical attention. The doctor I was working with at the time wasn't very familiar with handling large birds, so before we entered the exam room, I gave him a few quick pointers: "If the bird is in a cage, bring the whole cage or carrier to the back and I'll show you how to restrain him. If he's being held by the owner, grab a towel first, and I'll walk you through the proper technique."

We almost always have to restrain birds briefly in a towel to perform a physical exam, especially when treating wings or feet. If you own a bird and take it to the vet, you should expect this to happen. It keeps both the staff and the bird safe. Dr. F felt comfortable with the plan that we discussed and headed into the exam room.

He was in the exam room longer than I expected. When he finally reappeared through the treatment room door, he had a massive macaw perched on his arm, completely unrestrained, and a look of pure worry plastered across his face.

I wish I had a picture of that moment. The mix of comedy and concern is burned into my memory, I couldn't help but laugh. But once I got over that, I realized we had a loose, powerful bird in the hospital, and that was no laughing matter. I directed Dr. F into our in-house lab, a small, enclosed room where we could shut the door, contain the bird, and prevent him from flying off into our hospital.

Once inside the smaller room, Dr. F explained, "The owner said Travis was a really good bird, and that we shouldn't have any trouble. He told me we could examine him without restraint, then put the bird on my arm and told me to bring him back for treatment."

I raised a suspicious eyebrow. This was not an ideal setup. Dr. F continued, "The owner also told me that sometimes Travis starts biting, but only if he gets startled. If he's near your face and starts biting, you just have to say, 'Travis, please stop biting my face,' and he'll stop."

I laughed again, but this time nervously. Did he really expect me to believe that if this bird latched onto my nose or cheek with that enormous beak, I could politely ask him to stop and he would? I had serious doubts.

Travis didn't know us, he was in a strange environment, and he was already uncomfortable because of his injured toe. Everything about the situation told me he could easily lash out. His beak was strong enough to take off a finger or damage an eye. I wasn't about to gamble on the owner's method of "verbal persuasion."

So, we went back to proper, proven bird restraint. We wrapped Travis in a towel to immobilize his wings, then I used my index finger and thumb around his neck, applying upward pressure at the base of his beak to gently extend his head. This keeps the head and beak secure without putting pressure on the airway. It's a safe technique and the best way to prevent anyone from being bitten.

As it turned out, Travis was a remarkably cooperative macaw. Once restrained, he allowed us to examine him, tolerated the styptic powder we applied to stop his bleeding, and even went home with a small collar around his neck to prevent him from chewing at his injured foot.

He did wonderfully, but what stuck with me the most wasn't the medical outcome. It was the image of Dr. F walking in, bird perched on his arm, with that mix of panic and resignation on his face, and the unforgettable phrase: "Travis, please stop biting my face."

Chapter 4

Patients on the loose!

As an emergency doctor, you are always thinking about the worst-case scenario and trying to prevent it. Every once in a while, though, something will catch you off guard, a situation you were not expecting or anticipating. It happens to the best of us, so here is a little background and a story about such a situation.

Day by day at the veterinary hospital, patients pass each other in the hallways and treatment areas. Dog A may be headed to surgery while Dog B is on the way to get x-rays, so they cross paths, most often led by employees and almost always attached to leashes.

As friendly as many patients can be, there are several reasons why their behavior may change at the hospital. It is an unfamiliar environment, their owners are not around, they may not understand the commands we use, and they may be in pain. After all, there is always a reason why an animal is brought to the hospital. Their behavior is usually easy to read if you are accustomed to it, but it is not always predictable. The smells and sounds of a veterinary hospital are foreign to them, and many animals associate those smells with anxiety or discomfort. For example, if their only past visit was for a vaccination, that memory may leave them uneasy and expecting another unpleasant experience. They may anticipate that something bad is about to happen, a needle prick for a vaccination or a blood draw might be their only reference point. In many ways, the hospital is as scary for them as it can be for us.

It is also important to remember that animals only have a few ways to defend themselves or warn others that they are uncomfortable. Their first instinct is to move away from the threat, to leave the room or run, but at the hospital they usually cannot do that since we often restrain them with leashes, carriers, or gentle holds. When retreat is not possible, they rely on their next line of defense, verbal and visual cues such as growling, hissing, ears pinned back, or head lowered. While these signals often work with other animals and people, there are times when we still need to perform procedures they do not enjoy, even something as basic as a physical examination. If all else fails, they resort to their final method of defense, physical aggression through biting or scratching. Most of the time, these acts are quick and only used as a last resort, but as veterinarians and technicians, we must always be prepared.

We do our best to prevent such outcomes through a variety of techniques. Sometimes we have the luxury of moving slowly, giving the patient time to grow comfortable with us. We rely on proper restraint methods, often called "fear-free" techniques, and many times we use sedatives, pain medications, or anesthesia if we must perform something uncomfortable. This prevents them from having to resort to physical defense. For animals that are especially fearful or aggressive, we may need to use protective barriers like E-collars or muzzles to safely approach them. In our world, muzzles are not a sign of a bad animal, but simply a precaution, much like wearing oven mitts when handling hot pans.

Even with all these precautions, there are still moments when animals choose the more aggressive option. Despite our training, awareness, and restraint methods, bites and scratches do occasionally occur. While these injuries may seem minor compared to the risks in large animal medicine (like getting kicked by a horse), they can become serious if not managed quickly. In fact, bites and scratches are the most common type of workplace injury in small animal veterinary practice, and there are likely thousands of such cases every year across the country. Pictured in Figure 6 is a bite deterrent station from our hospital

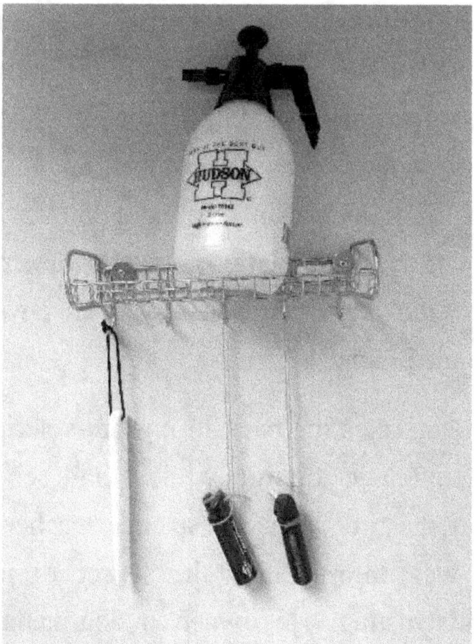

Figure 6

To help prevent injuries, we undergo annual safety training, and veterinarians, as well as many technicians, are vaccinated for rabies.

Our employers also keep us informed about the frequency of workplace injuries. Interestingly, the second most common injury in veterinary practice is not animal-related but back injuries, caused by constant lifting, stooping, bending, and moving.

We also take measures to prevent animal-on-animal injuries. One incident in particular stands out, which occurred in a hallway between exam rooms. Two clients exited their rooms at the same time, and when one door opened, a dog lunged and clamped down on another dog. The aggressor simply would not let go. It took every tool we had to separate them, and after that one event, we were forced to implement new protocols. We reviewed when exam room doors should be opened or closed, trained employees more thoroughly, and eventually installed bite-deterrent stations in all of our hospitals. At first, these bite stations seemed excessive, but anyone who has ever tried to break up a locked-in dog fight knows how difficult and dangerous it can be. The stations include deterrent sprays, water sprayers, noise makers, devices to pry open jaws, and even metal sheets to separate animals.

This incident takes me back to my pre-veterinary days, when I experienced a traumatic dog fight while in high school. It left a lasting impression. At the time, I had a science teacher named Mr. Gay, whose name was unfortunately the source of jokes, but he was intelligent and trusting. He owned a dog kennel in addition to teaching, likely to supplement his income. It was more than just a kennel, though, as he and his family also bred German Shepherds and trained them in Schutzhund, a German discipline meaning "protection dog." These dogs were trained in obedience, tracking, and protection work, much like police dogs. I often worked with them, sometimes playing the role of the "attacker" while wearing a large burlap bite sleeve. The dogs would chase me and tackle me by the'arm. It was thrilling, educational, and occasionally a little frightening.

Eventually, I began volunteering at the kennel to strengthen my veterinary school application, and later I worked there part-time. One weekend, while Mr. Gay and his family were away, I stayed at their house to care for the kenneled dogs. My morning routine went smoothly as I fed them, let them out, and cleaned their spaces. After finishing with the boarding building, I moved on to the smaller outdoor kennel where his German Shepherds were kept. Following instructions, I let them into the large fenced yard for exercise while I filled water buckets and prepared food.

At first, everything was normal. The dogs ran and played across several acres, enjoying their freedom. But within minutes, the calm shattered. I heard a growl, then the unmistakable sound of a dog fight. Before I could process what was happening, it erupted into chaos. More growls, barks, and yelps filled the air. I ran around the corner and was met with a horrifying sight: six German Shepherds locked in a full-on fight, teeth snapping, hair flying, and blood already visible on one of their heads. My heart pounded as panic set in. I had seen two dogs fight before, but never six at once. The scene was overwhelming, and I had no idea what to do.In retrospect, I am not sure if that fight broke out because I was not their usual caretaker, because I was preparing their food, or for some other unknown reason, since dog behavior is remarkably complex. Regardless, there I was in the middle of a massive dog brawl that I could not stop. It is not a common thing to be involved in such a situation, but it is terrifying.

The dogs were completely out of control. I yelled, screamed, clapped my hands, pushed, and shoved, but nothing changed. I thought about punching or kicking, but that is not in my nature. I grabbed two dogs by their collars and pulled with all my strength, managing to separate them for a brief second, but then they turned on me. I pulled my hands back just in time to avoid a nasty bite. I was petrified and had no idea what to do next. A friend had come with me that morning to help with the kennels, but he was inside the house and could not hear my screams. I was alone.

The struggle wore me down until I was in tears, shouting helplessly. Then I remembered the water buckets. Grabbing one filled with freezing cold water, it was early spring in Canada, I hurled it at the dogs. Thankfully, it was just enough to startle them, they briefly paused their attacks on each other and separated, long enough for me to "bark" their names at the top of my lungs and drive them back into their individual kennels. I slammed the doors shut and collapsed, exhausted and shaking.

Looking through the kennels, I saw that four of the dogs were bleeding. My heart sank as I realized the responsibility was mine, and they needed care immediately. Once I regained some composure, I called Mr. Gay and then the veterinarian. Bite wounds may appear minor on the surface, but they can hide severe damage beneath the skin, cause infection, and even lead to death.

Thankfully, Mr. Gay was understanding and did not hold me responsible. He knew I had done what I could do (and was told to do), and he knew canine behavior well. Four dogs needed veterinary treatment, but they healed over time. Still, the experience left me with a lifetime lesson: always do everything possible to prevent a multi-dog fight.

These days, I often joke that the hospital is no place for animals to make new animal friends. Even letting them sniff each other in such a stressful environment can trigger a dangerous incident.

Where was I headed with this story? Ah, yes, animal restraint. Even with our best efforts, animals occasionally slip out of our control. Dogs are usually easier since they arrive on leashes, but cats can be far more challenging. Even if they come in a carrier, we still have to coax them out, examine them, and return them inside.

Now and then, a cat will escape our grip and run loose in the clinic. Most of the time, we can corral them into a room or corner, but trouble arises if that space contains a fridge, x-ray machine, or other equipment they can hide behind, or under, or even inside of. I have seen cats disappear into ceiling tiles and even slip into the cavity between drywall. Neither was fun to resolve.

If a cat is every cornered in a hsoptal, they can become fractious (biting and swatting); we often use thick, bite-proof leather gloves to safely handle the cat in that situation, or we wrap them in a large, thick blanket or towel like a burrito. A heavy blanket can be surprisingly effective for restraining an angry feline.

But let me take another turn in this story. This one is not about a dog or a cat, but about a bird. One of the first questions we ask bird owners when they bring their pets in is whether the wings are clipped. Most pet birds have clipped wings, which involves trimming their large flight feathers so they cannot take off. They can still glide gently to the ground, much like a parachute, but they cannot launch themselves into sustained flight. Clipping wings is painless, much like trimming hair, and is done primarily for safety. A clipped bird that escapes a cage can be easily recaptured, while one with intact wings can quickly vanish into the sky (if outside) or up into the ceiling (if inside)...you've probably seen birds in the ceilings of large warehouse stores; now a veterinary hospital is not that big, but the challenge of recapturing a bird in that situation can be daunting.

In the veterinary setting, clipped wings also make handling safer. If a bird's wings are not clipped, we only open the cage in a fully enclosed room with no escape routes. A clipped bird will simply glide down, but a flighted bird can take off and circle indefinitely, making capture difficult. The risks of losing restraint are significant: injury to the bird, or worse, exposure to hospitalized dogs and cats, who are natural predators. A loose bird could also fly into kennels, disappear into high ceilings, or even escape through a door or window into the outdoors.

One day, a cockatiel came in whose wings had not been clipped. Sure enough, he slipped free and began flying around our ICU. I was in my office when I first heard someone shout, "Oh crap! Someone try and catch the bird!"

Moments later, I saw staff racing into the ICU armed with blankets and nets. I walked calmly into the chaos. Being an ER veterinarian, it takes a lot to rattle me, and I often serve as the voice of calm when panic sets in. Inside, the team was darting from corner to corner, chasing the bird as he happily flitted from one side of the ICU to the other.

Finally, someone pleaded, "Dr. Linklater, can you help us, please?!"

I stepped in and gave my first order: "Everyone calm down. Stop chasing him, you're only making him more anxious." My second instruction was to close all doors and kennel gates to contain the space. Once that was done, I walked to the middle of the ICU, raised my arm slowly, and held my index finger out sideways in the air, much like in Figure 7.

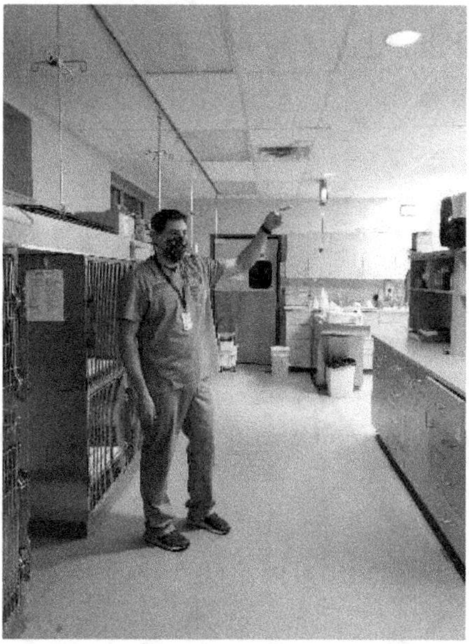

Figure 7

The staff stared at me in confusion. Then, the cockatiel launched from his perch, glided across the ICU, and landed gently on my finger.

I smiled, secured him in my hand, and carried him into a closed space for his examination.

You see, some birds are finger-trained, meaning they will willingly perch on an outstretched finger. Nobody else thought of that trick at the time, but it was simple and effective.

The cockatiel was unharmed and happy to have a safe perch to land on, and I was relieved to have him back under care without injury.

“Know your birds, people!” I said, walking out of the ICU with the bird in hand.

It turns out that day, one in the hand really is worth two in the bush.

Chapter 5

Dino the dinosaur

So my fiancée, now wife, and I are huge dinosaur fans. So much so that our wedding cake topper was a pair of T-rex dressed as a bride and groom, and one of our wedding gifts was the blow-up dinosaur costumes that became so popular around 2018.

I recall when we went to a movie theater to see the newest Jurassic World movie, the second one that has now been out for a few years, we left shaking our heads a little. You see, we may be dinosaur lovers, and I also love sci-fi, but some of the stuff in that movie was a little "out there," even for us. One of the characters in the movie described themselves as a "paleo-veterinarian," which is presumably a veterinarian for dinosaurs. We scoffed. Perhaps there is such a profession in the Jurassic Park universe, but unfortunately there is no such thing in the real world. We enjoyed the rest of the movie, but we scoffed again at the scene where one of the dinosaurs had been shot. In typical movie fashion, they pulled the bullet out with hemostats, dropped it into a metal pan with a loud clink, and declared that the poor dinosaur was going to be fine. Again, pure fiction, and I shook my head.

That scene was wrong on so many levels. In my career, I've had the unfortunate task of treating many animals which have been shot and have bullets inside them. It's actually not that uncommon; we see several gunshot victims each year. We almost never go after or retrieve the bullet unless it is causing a specific problem. The risk of surgery and cutting through multiple layers of tissue or organ to retrieve a small metal fragment is simply not worth it when the fragment isn't causing harm. Most of the time, attempting removal will cause more damage than leaving the bullet in place.

There are exceptions of course. If the bullet happens to be lodged in a particularly dangerous location, like the spinal canal, or if it is actively causing a major problem, then yes, we will attempt to retrieve it. But in the vast majority of cases, bullets and other small metal fragments are left where they are. Think about people and animals who undergo orthopedic surgery for a broken bone or hip replacement; they are often left with large pieces of metal hardware inside their bodies. On a smaller scale, dental fillings used to be made of metal. Most metals, even lead, generally do not cause problems when embedded in tissue. Lead only becomes an issue if it is ingested and absorbed in the stomach. Metals like steel and titanium do not get absorbed at all.

Back to that Jurassic Park movie, I was actually intrigued by the scene where they gave a blood transfusion from a T-rex to a Velociraptor. As fake as that sounded, there was actually some truth and science behind it. Probably not the safest thing to collect blood from a T-rex, although it was sedated in the film, and I cannot imagine how easy it would be to locate a vein and get a needle into it. But xenotransfusion, when blood is taken from one species and given to another, is in fact real.

Xenotransfusions are occasionally performed in veterinary medicine, though they are extremely rare. Most transfusions occur within the same species, dog to dog or cat to cat, and usually the same blood type is required, especially in cats. You might recall the tortoise transfusion I mentioned earlier. However, in rare cases, blood of a certain species is very scarce or not available at all. This happens most often with cats. Dogs, being larger and generally more cooperative, can be trained to donate blood. Cats, on the other hand, make poor donors; they don't sit still, only small volumes can be taken, and eventually they grow to despise the process. Cats also only have two blood types, A and B. Type B cats are rare (at least in the US), and giving the wrong blood type can be fatal because cats often have pre-formed antibodies against the other type.

Because of this, cat blood is especially scarce and valuable. There are published cases of veterinarians giving dog blood to cats in emergencies. This is xenotransfusion. I have not done this myself, but I have come close several times, and many of my colleagues have as well. When the alternative is death from blood loss or severe anemia, the risk of giving a foreign-species transfusion may occasionally be worth taking. Still, it is considered a last-ditch effort, done with extreme caution, and in cats it can only be attempted once. Within days, they will develop antibodies against dog blood, making further transfusions impossible.

Now, I've digressed a bit into transfusions, but this story is really about dinosaurs, or at least their modern-day relatives: lizards.

Yes, dinosaurs once ruled the world, but today much smaller lizards inhabit nearly every warm environment across the globe. Some of the larger lizard species are quite successful and likely resemble dinosaurs in many ways, such as crocodiles and Komodo dragons.

There is also a booming pet lizard industry. Iguanas and bearded dragons are the most common, but we do see the occasional monitor lizard, gecko, or uromastyx at our hospital. There is even a veterinary certification in reptile medicine available under the American Board of Veterinary Practice. Specialized reptile and amphibian interest groups also exist. While there are no true dinosaur veterinarians, the closest modern equivalent to a "paleo-veterinarian" would be a veterinarian who specializes in reptiles. Many veterinarians, myself included, practice on exotic species like reptiles. And this brings me to the story of Dino.

Dino is a five-year-old Savannah monitor. At my practice, more than 95 percent of our patients are dogs and cats. We do occasionally treat rabbits, small mammals, birds, reptiles, and other species, including, on rare occasions, a monkey. Much to the chagrin of my coworkers, when we receive an emergency call about an exotic pet, we usually say yes if it seems like a true emergency. We are always honest with owners, explaining that we are not exotic species specialists, although more recently we added a team of exotic-only veterinarians, including a specialist. Their pets will need follow-up care with someone experienced in their species, but we still want to provide a place for owners to turn in emergencies. Our hospital is certified as a Veterinary Emergency and Critical Care Society (VECCS) Level I emergency center, and part of that certification involves being able to see exotics on an emergency basis.

So, we got the call. Dino the Savannah monitor had eaten a piece of Styrofoam, like a packing peanut. On its own, that might not have been too bad, since Styrofoam is not toxic. But the piece was large enough to sit in his stomach without dissolving or passing into the intestines. This meant it could either obstruct his stomach or reduce the amount of nutrients he could absorb. Unfortunately, this was not one of the dissolving cornstarch-based peanuts. I recommended Dino be evaluated by our emergency service.

He came in, and our technicians were reluctant to touch a three-foot monitor lizard. He glared with beady eyes and flicked his forked tongue at us. He spent some time in the hospital while we collected his history, and after a while I could see the nurses warming up to him. I actually thought Dino seemed kind of cute. You'll see there are several pictures of him (Figures 8-11), which we'll get to shortly.

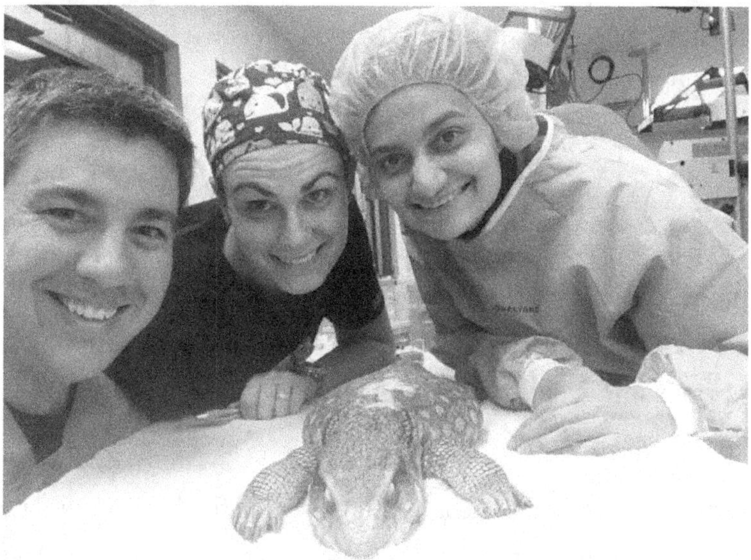

Figure 8

I've dealt with many lizards before, but not a monitor. There are certainly things to be cautious about, mainly their razor-sharp claws. Their teeth can also be dangerous, capable of ripping tissue easily. To ensure our safety, we donned gloves before handling him and performing a physical exam. Unlike many of the exotic species we see, Dino was in excellent shape, with good coloring and body condition. Sadly, many exotic pets arrive in poor health, usually due to a lack of education on their care rather than intentional neglect. Dino, however, looked great.

From his history, we learned he had already vomited three pinky mice he had been fed earlier that day, and he had been lethargic for a few hours before coming in. This was unusual for just having eaten a Styrofoam peanut. Knowing this, we discussed options with the owner: x-rays, using an endoscope to try to remove the object, or going directly to surgery. I was reluctant to offer surgery, as no one on duty had performed surgery nor anesthesia on a lizard before. I had assisted years ago, but it had been a long time.

The owners, after much debate, decided they wanted to try the endoscopy, or "scope," to remove the piece of Styrofoam from Dino's stomach. I was comfortable with scoping, as you probably know by this point from the various things I've removed from animals. The owners were on board, and I agreed to perform the procedure, but not before consulting both textbook references and a colleague about lizard anesthesia.

Lizard anesthesia is not particularly difficult. We can induce anesthesia with intramuscular injections, intubate them by placing a tube in the trachea just as we would with a cat, dog, or person, and then give gas anesthesia. But lizards present unique challenges. Yes, we would literally have to monitor the monitor.

When a lizard is under anesthesia, its heart rate can drop so low that it may beat only once per minute, and its respiratory rate is not much better. Regular breaths are necessary for patients under anesthesia because they help keep them anesthetized with inhalant gas. Other monitoring tools, like blood pressure and ECG, are nearly useless on reptiles. My technician, who would be monitoring anesthesia during the procedure, was understandably hesitant. She enjoyed treating exotic species but knew the risks, and although not completely comfortable, she was skilled and willing to tackle this challenge with me.

After inducing anesthesia and inserting the breathing tube (Figure 9), Dino did surprisingly well. We passed the scope into his stomach, located the foreign body, and tried to remove it with a small pair of graspers. But it would not move past a small brown object in his stomach. Suddenly, the Styrofoam slipped off the graspers, and we struggled to move it into his esophagus. During endoscopy, the stomach must be inflated with air so there is space between the camera tip and the object we're viewing.

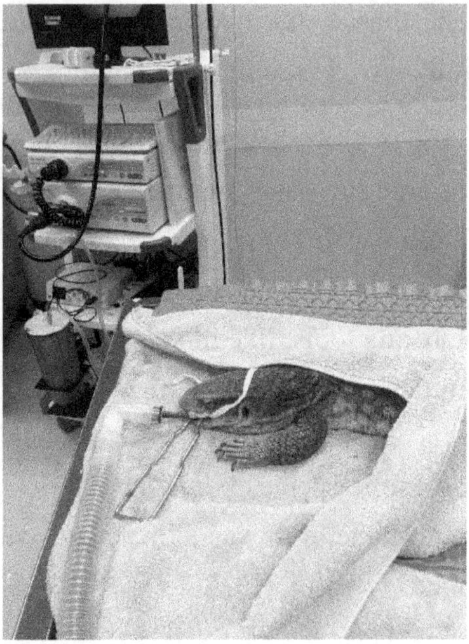

Figure 9

Imagine pressing your finger against a camera lens, you cannot see clearly until you move the finger away and create perspective. The same principle applies to endoscopy. Unfortunately, Dino's stomach never inflated well, which made visualizing anything extremely difficult.

We went back down the esophagus with the scope, but inflation remained a problem. Then I noticed a hole, not a very big one. Unsure what I was seeing, I advanced the scope through it and suddenly found myself looking at ribs and blood vessels. This meant I was in the coelomic cavity, the abdominal space outside of the gastrointestinal tract. That was bad news. It meant there was a hole in his stomach, which would allow food and fluid to leak into the body cavity and cause a life-threatening infection if not repaired.

My heart absolutely sank. The "hole" I identified was a gastric (stomach) rupture, meaning that without surgery, poor Dino would die. Not only was I devastated for him, but I also worried that I might have caused the damage. I had only participated in one lizard surgery before in my career, and now I was facing an open procedure with this monitor lizard. On top of that, I didn't know if the owners would even agree to such an expensive surgery. I was literally sweating.

After a moment, I collected myself and reviewed the situation. Dino was stable under anesthesia. I examined my equipment and technique and became fairly confident I had *not* caused the rupture. How did I know? Several reasons. First, there was no blood around the edges of the hole, which suggested the wound was not fresh. Second, it is nearly impossible to rupture a healthy stomach with an endoscope unless the tissue is already diseased. The final reason would reveal itself later. Despite my anxiety, as the leader of the team I had to remain calm. Eight people had gathered to watch the "really cool lizard scope," and the room fell silent as we realized the gravity of the situation.

I called the owners. They wanted nothing but the best for their boy. I explained the options: surgery with me, an "inexperienced" lizard surgeon, or referral to the veterinary school, which would delay surgery at least 12 to 24 hours, not a good option for Dino. To my relief (for Dino), but my anxiety (for me!), they wanted me to move forward and said they had confidence in me.

We also discussed possible causes of the rupture. The owner mentioned Dino had fallen about a foot from his perch the day before, though I would have expected bruising if that were the cause. He also mentioned feeding large raw shrimp, and I wondered if the sharp tail scutes could have punctured the stomach. Another possibility was the piece of wood we later discovered in his stomach.

For Dino's surgery out came the textbooks again. I reviewed lizard anatomy, anesthesia protocols, surgical techniques, and aftercare. I relayed the plan to my technician, who, though just as anxious as I was, stayed cool and prepared for surgery.

Two important things are drilled into veterinary students about lizard surgery. First, reptiles do not have a diaphragm separating chest from abdomen; instead, they have one continuous cavity called the coelomic cavity. Second, a large vein runs down the middle of the ventral abdomen, which must be avoided at all costs during surgery.

Dino was still under anesthesia and moved to the surgery suite, given pain medication, prepped for surgery, and I scrubbed in, sweating under my cap and mask.

To my relief, things went as smoothly as they possibly could. I made the incision into his coelomic cavity, located the hole in the stomach right at the junction with the esophagus, and sutured it closed, making sure it did not leak. Then I created a controlled incision into a healthy part of the stomach and removed the foreign material. Remarkably, Dino was doing well under anesthesia, there was minimal contamination in the coelomic cavity from the gastric rupture. "Doing well" under anesthesia for a lizard means we were breathing for him and watching for a heartbeat every 30 seconds or so, which is daunting compared to mammal patients.

When I opened the stomach (Figure 10), one word came to mind: disgusting. Inside were seven partially digested, slimy, foul-smelling pinky mice, along with the styrofoam, shrimp tails, and a medium-sized piece of wood. After removing the contents, we lavaged the cavity, checked the sutures, and closed him up. I even put a couple of the mice back inside his stomch to provide him with some nutrition for recovery. Ultimately, we determined the rupture was chronic, likely caused by the shrimp scutes or the wood lodged sideways in his stomach, which weakened the wall over time. The endoscope had simply revealed the injury, which explained why he had been unwell even before eating the Styrofoam.

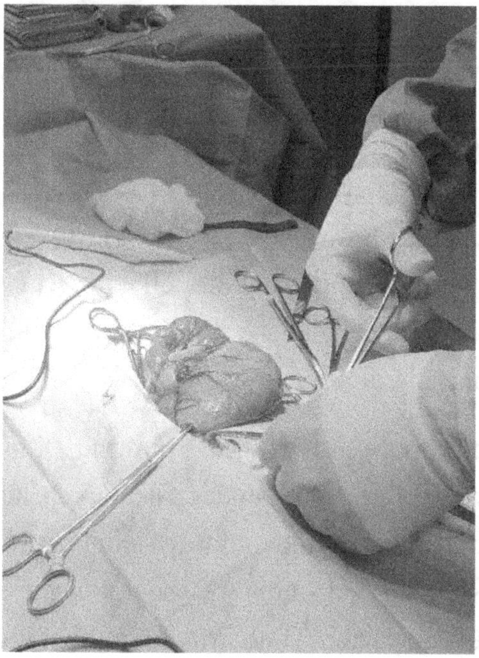

Figure 10

Closing a reptile's abdomen is no easy task. In mammals, we close in three layers: the abdominal wall, the subcutaneous tissue, and then the skin, which provides security. Reptiles are different. Their tough scales invert on themselves, leaving little substance to stitch together. The abdomen must be closed in one perfect layer, with zero room for error.

Once Dino's scales were sutured, we discontinued anesthesia. Now came the next challenge: recovery. Most patients lose body heat under anesthesia because of the cold surgical tables, body cavity exposure, metal instruments, and drugs that impair thermoregulation. For reptiles, temperature is everything. Cold slows their metabolism, and recovery can take hours. But overheating is equally dangerous. We had to get it just right. Dino even had an old skin burn from improper heat support at another hospital in the past, so we were careful not to repeat that!

By now it was 3 a.m., four hours past my shift, but I had to ensure everything was in place before leaving. Records could wait until morning, the patient was always the priority. Dino was slow to recover, and I finally tapped out at 3:30 a.m., leaving a plan with the attending DVM and technicians. But not before taking a team photo with our "monitor lizard miracle"

The next morning, I was thrilled to find Dino still lethargic but doing fairly well. We had him under a heat lamp, and one of our techs had a brilliant idea: it was the middle of summer, so why not take him outside to bask in natural sunlight? The effect was miraculous. Three 30-minute sessions later, Dino was alert, flicking his tongue, and moving around.

We all "oohed and aahed" over him. Most of the other vets congratulated me on the accomplishment and bravery, compliments we rarely give one another, so they meant a lot.

And then the amazing happened. We offered Dino food, and not only did he eat, but he asked for more (Figure 11). We were overjoyed to call the owner and let him know Dino could go home with postoperative medications and careful monitoring.

We will be talking about the monitor lizard surgery at our hospital for years. In the end, it turned out to be a truly great day.

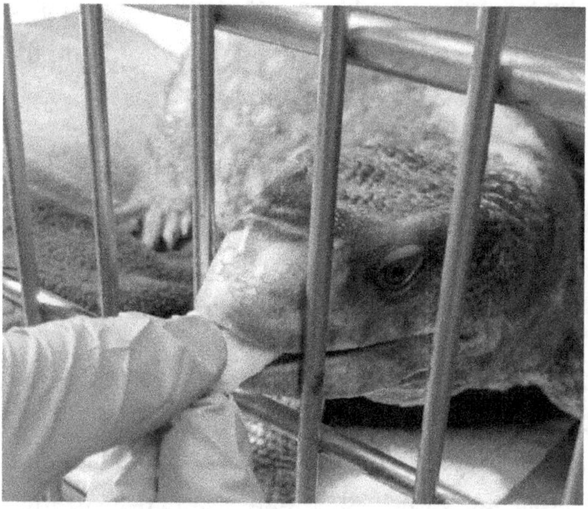

Figure 11

Chapter 6

The similarity between sharks and chickens

So, if you were ever a dinosaur fan in the modern age (post-Jurassic Park), you are probably aware of the similarities drawn between dinosaurs and birds, and perhaps that was the evolutionary path they went down, but I bet no one ever told you there are a few similarities between sharks and chickens!

I'll confess, I haven't spent much time around sharks. I've visited aquariums, sure, and I've spent time with dolphins, beluga whales, sea lions and more, but not many sharks. As I've alluded to before, I grew up in the landlocked province of Saskatchewan, so there wasn't much exposure to aquariums. Like many people who love animals, including veterinarians, I did make a trip to South Africa where I spent a few weeks enjoying the culture, sights and sounds of another country. It was one of the most memorable trips of my life and I hope to go back someday. While I was there, of course I had to take the opportunity to go diving with great whites, maybe a story for another time. It was an incredible experience and one I highly recommend. Sadly, some orcas drove away the great whites in the late 2010s, devastating the shark tourism industry in Cape Town, so definitely do some research before you go!

At some point during my interest in sharks, probably while watching Shark Week on The Discovery Channel, I learned that if you turn sharks upside down, you can lull them to sleep. Turns out the exact same thing is true for chickens! I don't remember where I first learned this about chickens, but it is true.

One evening at the emergency hospital, we got a call about a chicken that had suffered trauma, and the owners wanted it treated. I confirmed with our front desk that I was willing to see the case. We suspected the poor bird, who was showing signs of abdominal pain, needed radiographs (x-rays). To get clear radiographs of most birds, they often need to be sedated or fully anesthetized so we can position their body correctly. That comes with risk, and we try to avoid anesthesia whenever possible.

I spoke with the owners about taking radiographs and they agreed. I went back into the treatment area and put in the orders to anesthetize the chicken and proceed with x-rays. My technicians saw the order and asked if there was anything else to do. Somewhere in the back of my mind, through the cobwebs of stored knowledge, came a revelation.

"Of course!" I shouted. "We don't have to anesthetize her, we can just hypnotize her!" My technicians looked at me like I'd lost it. "Huh?"

Yes, you can actually hypnotize chickens so they will sit still long enough to get an x-ray. I don't recall exactly where I learned this, but I knew it was true. It's a simple technique, though I'm still not sure how or why it works. You hold the chicken snugly with its wings wrapped against its body, then rotate it onto its back. Some people suggest twirling a finger in front of the beak or drawing a line on the table starting near the beak and moving away. I'm not sure how effective the second part is, but it seemed harmless enough to try, so we did.

I bundled up the chicken, rolled her onto her back, and while an assistant twirled her finger in front of the beak, she stayed still long enough for us to take the x-ray. Figure 12 shows me and an assistant performing the technique after the x-rays, teaching the rest of the staff how to do it. I even recorded a video for future reference.

The x-rays turned out to be pretty normal, so we started her on some supportive medications and sent her home that night. I'm told she did well.

And now you know the similarity between sharks and chickens!

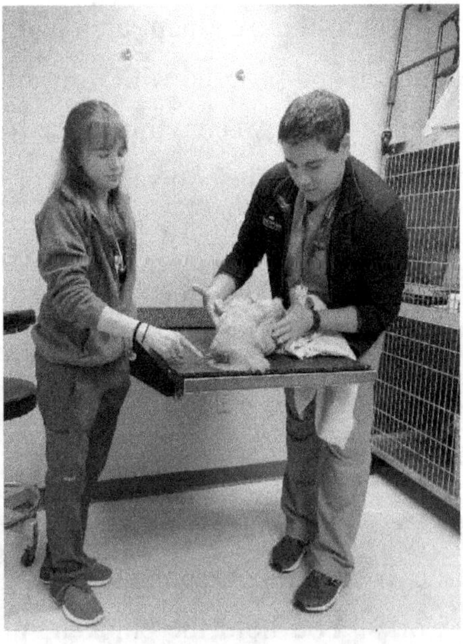

Figure 12

Section 6 - Ouch! That has GOT to Hurt!

Chapter 1

The Twisted Tie

Well, here are some uncomfortable topics to discuss, so let's just call it out. The first two stories in this section are going to talk about animal reproductive parts and habits. Get comfortable with it, because it might feel a little awkward.

Believe me, when you go through veterinary school and learn about things like how to collect sperm from different animals, it gets uncomfortable quickly. Most male animals need some kind of female stimulation, like a dog in heat, to get them excited, and then require some manual stimulation to "finish the job" so that semen can be collected, examined and stored for later use in artificial insemination. This is done for many reasons, usually to "overbreed" animals with desirable characteristics, so those traits are passed on. Maybe a golden retriever has a particular look, or a bull's offspring produce more milk. Whatever the case, artificial insemination is a common practice in veterinary medicine.

This is not something I do in my practice, but plenty of veterinarians do. My exposure was mostly in veterinary school, and these lessons are not easily forgotten. I vividly remember in herd health and reproductive classes, our professor manually stimulating a male dog. The act was very similar to masturbation, except a person was doing it to a dog, and that image does not leave your mind easily. With horses, things work a little differently. They can perform the manual part themselves, but with some precautions. First, handlers need to keep a safe distance so no one gets hurt, and second, instead of breeding a female, the stallion is encouraged to mount a dummy. His penis is then guided into an AV, or artificial vagina, so the semen can be collected. Bulls, however, "take the cake" for the strangest method. For bovine species, we often use an electro-ejaculator, a metal, rocket-shaped device a little thicker than a baguette. It is inserted into the rectum and slowly worked until it stimulates the bull to ejaculate. It is safe and effective, but to an outsider, it looks quite harsh. I have only seen each of these procedures a few times in my career, and although awkward, they are simply part of biology. Fun tasks for veterinarians and farm workers, right?

Hopefully that gets the discomfort out of the way, because now we can move on to some stories. For those who do not know about "the tie," a quick explanation is needed. When dogs mate, the base of the male's penis swells to a point that it becomes stuck inside the female for several minutes. This is nature's way of ensuring sperm remain in place to increase the chance of pregnancy. The swelling is so significant that the two dogs are literally locked together for a short time. Because the mating position cannot be sustained for long, the male usually swings a leg over the female, twisting slightly, and the two remain stuck butt to butt until the swelling goes down and they separate.

This natural process has, of course, led to some amusing conversations in veterinary clinics, like imagining how awkward things would be if humans had a similar arrangement.

At the hospital, we usually get a few calls each year from panicked owners whose dogs are stuck together after mating. Most of the time, we tell them to wait a few minutes, and the tie will resolve naturally. On one occasion, however, the owners waited, called back, tried our suggestions of water, a cool washcloth, or even a gentle dip in a cool bath, but the dogs remained stuck. After nearly an hour, they brought them into the clinic. By then the dogs were relatively calm, but obviously uncomfortable, especially if either one tried to move.

Both dogs were brought into the treatment area, the male wearing an innocent "I didn't do anything wrong" expression, and the female with a look that could only be translated as "this is your fault, and I'm furious." His penis was literally lodged inside her vagina, and no amount of lubrication or local anesthetic seemed to help.
See Figure 1.

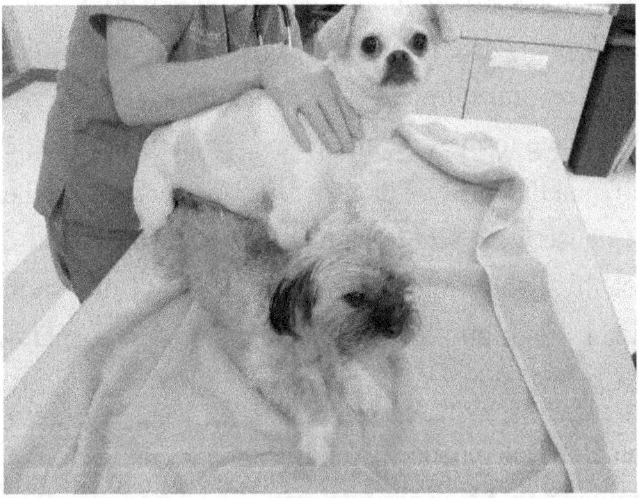

Figure 1

The question became, which dog do we sedate? Both the male and female were contributing to the swelling, so either could have been the target. Sedating both was an option, but came with additional risks. One of the sedatives we sometimes use, acepromazine, carries a rare side effect called priapism, where the penis remains permanently extruded. It happens most commonly in horses, but has been reported in other species as well, so it was not our first choice. We opted for other medications.

The female was becoming increasingly agitated, so she was sedated first. Once she was relaxed, we tried again with lubrication, but it still didn't work. Eventually we sedated the male as well, and after more lubrication and careful manipulation, we were finally able to separate the two.

Both dogs were undoubtedly sore and uncomfortable. For reference, the next image we captured was quite graphic, showing the male dog's penis after separation. See Figure 2. It was swollen, bruised, and rotated almost 90 degrees clockwise. We applied cooling wraps and sent both dogs home on anti-inflammatory and pain medications. They recovered well within a few days.As for whether the mating was successful, I never did find out.

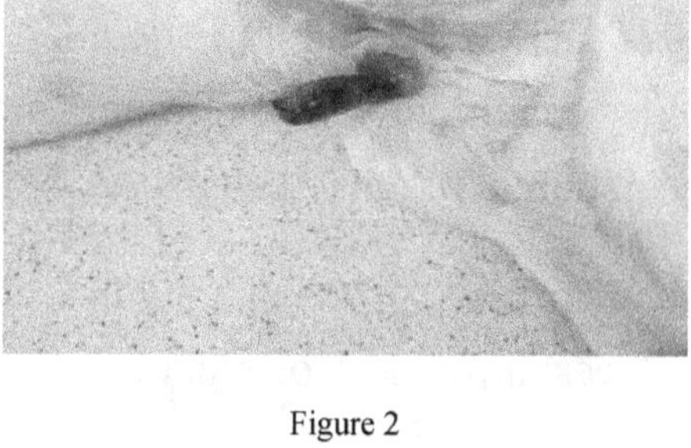

Figure 2

Chapter 2

T-rex the chicken

Well, I'm sure you've figured it out by this point that I primarily treat dogs and cats. We do get some exotic species at our hospital, and once in a while, we see a few farm animals. Although the hospital where I've spent most of my career was located in suburban Wisconsin, you're never too far from farmland, hobby farms, and even cities that allow backyard chickens (the same is true where I now practice outside of Denver).

One night, we received a call about a chicken that was bleeding from her head, and the owners wanted to bring her in. It doesn't take much blood loss for any bird to reach a life-threatening state, so of course, we advised the owners to apply pressure to the area immediately and head in to the hospital as soon as possible.

When the chicken arrived, she was immediately triaged and taken to our treatment area. It's hospital policy that any patient presenting with a life-threatening condition is called as a STAT and taken immediately to the STAT triage area for assessment by a doctor. Life-threatening issues include breathing difficulties, blood loss, shock, seizures, and other conditions requiring intervention within minutes of arrival, or the patient's life may be at risk.

This was one instance where I couldn't change the patient's name. For some reason, owners of chickens always choose unique names for chickens. Over the years, we've seen Beatrice, Q-tip, and many others. This chicken's name was T-Rex. I never asked why, but T-Rex turned out to be an amazingly friendly bird. Most chickens are fairly easy to handle, and she was no exception.

During her physical exam, we didn't find much wrong aside from a large laceration on her comb that exposed part of her cranium. Otherwise, she seemed stable and in good spirits. The next step was to discuss treatment options with her owner. What she really needed was to have her comb and open wound sutured closed, which isn't a particularly complicated procedure. However, T-Rex would have to be anesthetized for it.

I need to back up for a moment and explain one of our hospital policies. Anytime a patient is scheduled for anesthesia, we always ask for a resuscitation code. This means that, in the unlikely event of a cardiac or respiratory arrest, we clarify whether the owners would like us to perform CPR. In veterinary medicine, there are typically three options: full CPR including opening the chest, known as a Green Code; full CPR without opening the chest, known as a Yellow Code; and finally, a Do Not Resuscitate order, also known as a Red Code. For birds, a Green Code isn't usually an option, so the choice is simply between performing CPR or not.

I had a detailed conversation with T-Rex's owner about the risks of anesthesia in birds. They face a higher risk of cardiac arrest compared to dogs or cats, and their outcomes following CPR are generally poor. When I discussed CPR with T-Rex's owner, she gasped, placed her hand over her chest, and said, "Why would anyone ***not*** do CPR on their chicken?" I absolutely loved that response! I chuckled because very few owners would actually choose to do CPR on a pet chicken. Most would opt for the Do Not Resuscitate option. But from that moment, I knew she truly loved her chicken and was willing to do whatever it took.

We gave T-Rex some pain medication and attempted to use local anesthesia so we could close the wound without putting her fully under, but she wouldn't tolerate it. Eventually, we decided she needed full general anesthesia to complete the procedure. A simple "gas mask" induction worked quickly, and soon she was sedated enough for me to begin the repair.

As it turned out, I had to remove a large portion of her comb—about two-thirds—to close the wound properly and ensure it would heal without complications. Figure 3-A shows T-rex when she was sedated with a large, bruised portion of her comb that had lost its blood supply. Figure 3-B, shows T-rex after the damaged portion of the comb was removed. Figure 4 shows the portion of the comb that had to be removed.The result gave T-Rex a noticeably smaller comb and a new, distinctive profile.

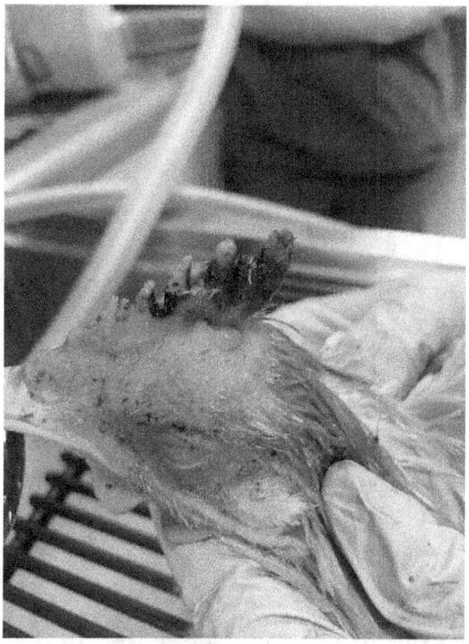

Figure 3-A

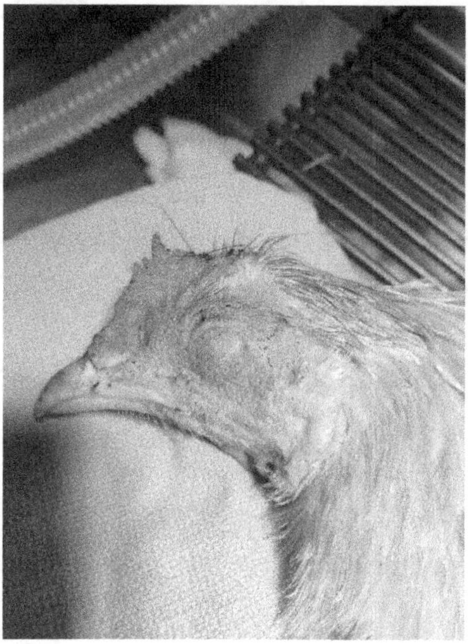

Figure 3-B

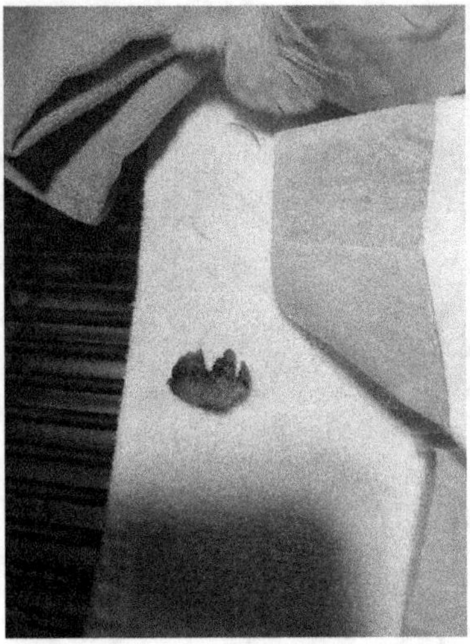

Figure 4

T-Rex was able to go home later that night, no worse for wear. About ten days later, she returned to have her sutures removed. Her head wound had healed beautifully, and her owners were very appreciative of our efforts to help save their bird.

You can see pictures of me with T-Rex in Figure 5, looking quite happy about her recovery from anesthesia. This was one of those times I learned never to judge what people are willing to do for their pets based on the species.

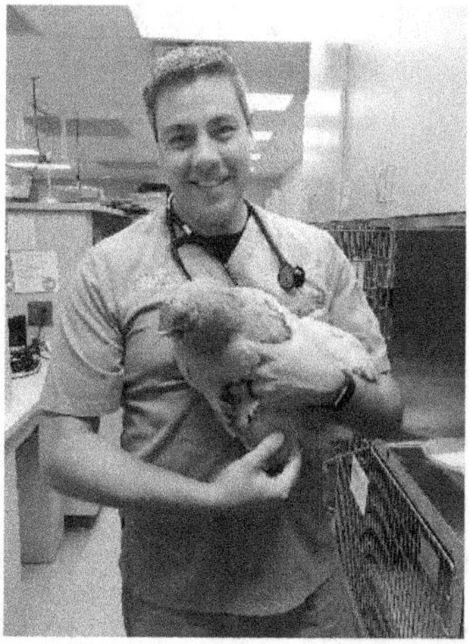

Figure 5

Later that year, a Christmas card arrived at the hospital from T-Rex's family (Figure 6). I absolutely had to include it in this book because it remains one of the most wonderful cards I've ever received. Inside were some heartfelt comments about the care we provided, and on the front was a custom picture of T-Rex—you can tell it's her because of her small comb—running around their yard wearing a red holiday scarf. I have never been more proud of having treated a pet bird than I was that day.

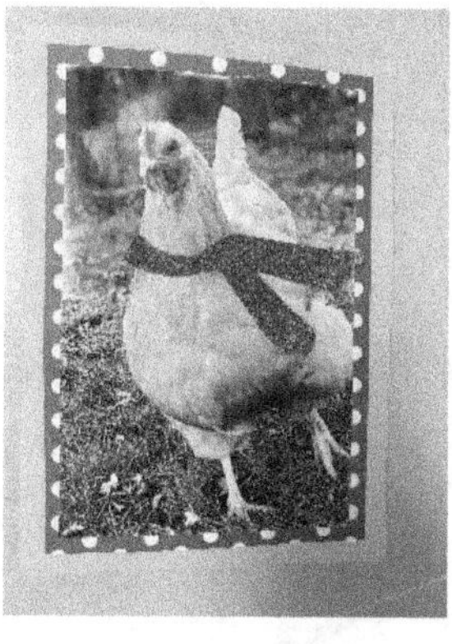

Figure 6

Chapter 3

The most "Wisconsin" Triage Ever!

I call this next story *"The Most Wisconsin Triage Ever"* because it includes so many elements that are uniquely Wisconsin. Since moving to Colorado, I've promised myself that one day I'll share *"The Most Colorado Triage Ever"* as well!

One late evening in the middle of winter, an elderly Golden Retriever was triaged at our hospital. The case was called as a STAT because the patient had sustained trauma, meaning there was a potential life-threatening issue and we needed to assess her immediately. When the older Golden Retriever was brought into the treatment area, it was immediately clear that her right forelimb was fractured—and it was an open fracture. The skin was torn, exposing the bone underneath. Figure 7 shows a picture of the forelimb with exposed bone, and Figure 8 shows the radiograph we later took.

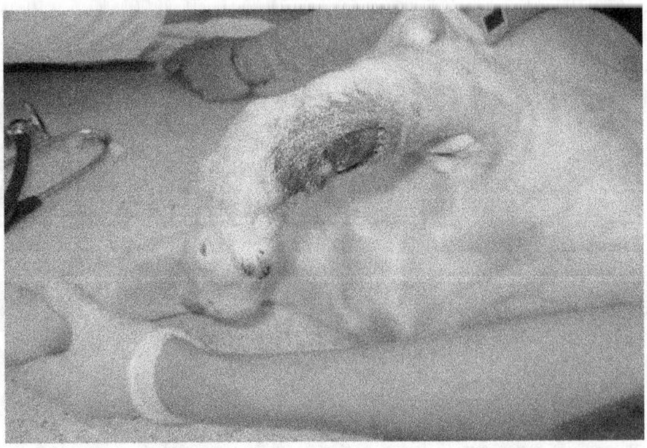

Figure 7

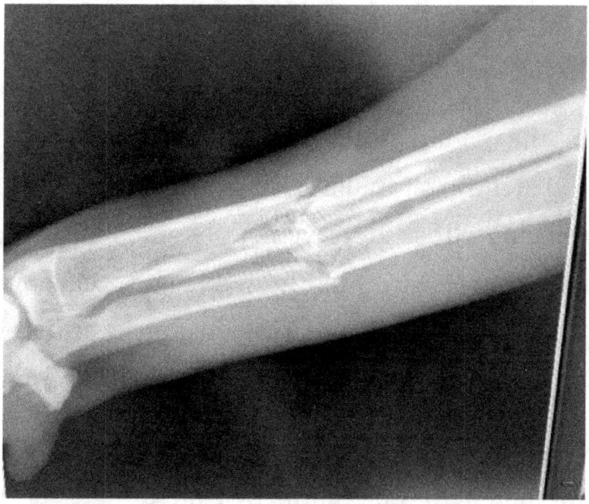

Figure 8

We immediately administered pain medication and applied a temporary bandage to limit further injury while gathering more information from the owners about how they wanted to proceed. Through it all, this lovely dog kept wagging her tail.

So, why do I call this the most Wisconsin triage ever? It's because of the circumstances surrounding the dog's injury. When we went into the examination room to gather more details from the owner—what we call taking the *history*—we asked the owner about what had happened, what the surrounding circumstances were, and whether there were any underlying health issues we should be aware of before moving forward with treatment.

We found ourselves speaking with the dog's female owner, who looked rather upset. Her face was flushed, and when we asked if any other family members needed to be consulted, she immediately said, "Absolutely not. My husband caused this accident, and we're paying for whatever our dog needs." It was quite clear she wasn't very happy with her husband at that moment.

Given the nature of the injury, we could tell the dog had experienced significant trauma. Most of the time, such fractures are caused by being struck by a vehicle—something we abbreviate as HBC (Hit by car)—or by a fall from a height. But as we asked more questions, we learned that this Golden Retriever had actually been struck by a snowmobile.

Now, snowmobiles themselves aren't unique to Wisconsin—they're common across the northern United States and Canada (and certainly around the world too!)—but the *reasons* behind this particular snowmobile accident were very Wisconsin-specific.

Unfortunately, it's quite common in northern Wisconsin for people to spend winter evenings snowmobiling from bar to bar. Just like driving a car under the influence, operating a snowmobile while intoxicated is illegal, but since riders often stick to back roads, ditches, and farm fields, it's not easily enforced by local officials. Still, as a responsible adult, I'd strongly advise against it. Snowmobiles are powerful machines that can travel at high speeds, and when you're navigating wooded areas, hitting a tree is a real risk. I actually owned a snowmobile myself at one point and even had a minor accident—which resulted in a fracture of my collarbone—and I can assure you, there was no alcohol involved in that one!

Now, what else is very Wisconsin-specific? I'd say beer, cheese, and the Packers. As it turns out, the owner of the snowmobile had been bar hopping, drinking beer, and the final stop of the night happened to be a cheese sampling party that coincided with a Packers game. And that's why I call this event *"The Most Wisconsin Triage Ever"* at our hospital.

That night, we cleaned and dressed the wound, administered pain medications and antibiotics, and closely monitored her vital signs, which remained stable. Within forty-eight hours, she underwent surgery with one of our orthopedic surgeons to repair the fracture. Although her recovery took several weeks, she healed beautifully and was soon doing very well.

Chapter 4

The Trifecta of Tongue Twister Torture Tales

There are so many things that can happen to tongues, oh boy! As I discussed in one of my previous stories, there are limited ways in which animals can explore their environment: sound, sight, smell, and often taste. Many dogs and cats explore their surroundings through taste. Sometimes those tastes are harmless, and sometimes they're delicious. However, there are times when those tastes can be downright dangerous, and you might never expect some of the situations that occur because of it. The following are a few instances where pets used their tongues when they probably should have thought twice.

The first story involves a cat who really wanted to help improve the household environment. As many of you know, animals often bring a certain odor with them. Try as we might—with grooming, Febreze, regular cleaning of litter boxes, and more—the smell tends to linger, particularly around the litter area for cat owners. Animals may think they're doing a great job grooming themselves, but for most of us, it doesn't quite meet our standards. So, we humans try all sorts of ways to improve how our homes smell: flowers, incense, more Febreze, scented candles (a big favorite at our house), and sometimes even potpourri.

Most people don't know that potpourri is actually quite toxic to dogs and cats, both in its liquid and dry forms. Potpourri contains many alkalinizing agents, such as essential oils, which can cause serious chemical burns to the tongue, esophagus, and stomach of animals. Most pets avoid it because the scent is so strong—what smells nice to us can be overwhelming to them. But for some animals, or perhaps just certain curious individuals, that curiosity gets the better of them. They investigate with a sniff, and sometimes, unfortunately, with a lick. So here's a word of caution: if you have cats or dogs and enjoy potpourri, you may want to reconsider or at least keep it well out of reach.

One young cat approached a bowl of potpourri while her owners were out. When they returned, they found her drooling profusely and pawing at her face. She was lethargic, hiding, and not interested in eating, so they rushed her to the clinic. During our physical exam, we noticed mild abdominal discomfort, a slightly elevated temperature, and heavy drooling. Around her lips, there was crusted debris, and when we examined her mouth (shown in Figure 9), we saw that the edges of her tongue were raw and red. The small abrasive papillae that give cat tongues' their rough texture had sloughed off around the edges. I can only imagine how painful that must have been, and of course, she wasn't going to want to eat for a while. And if that's what we could see in her mouth, imagine what her esophagus and stomach looked like.

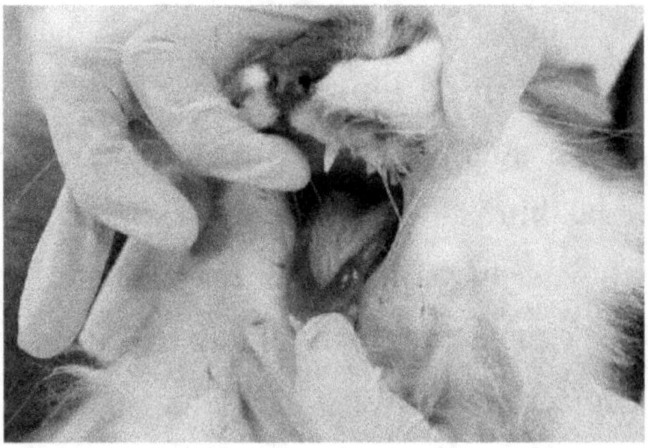

Figure 9

She required intensive supportive care until the swelling and inflammation improved. We hospitalized her for about a day and a half to provide pain relief, fluids, and medications to help heal her tongue, esophagus, and stomach. Thankfully, she recovered well, but we came close to having to place a temporary feeding tube. Cats that go without food for several days risk developing hepatic lipidosis, or fatty liver disease, which can be life-threatening. That, however, is a story for another day.

The next tongue twisting case was less about curiosity and more a consequence of disease. This involved an older terrier who had previously undergone surgery to remove a facial tumor. During the procedure, part of a nerve that supplied sensation to portions of her face had to be removed. Although she recovered well from the surgery, it likely left part of her tongue with altered sensation or tingling. Animals generally don't tolerate tingling well, and she ended up chewing on her own tongue. Figure 10 shows the damage she caused. Because of this, she needed to have a significant portion of her tongue surgically removed the next day. Interestingly, dogs can still eat and drink quite well even if more than half of their tongue is removed—a fact that surprises many people! She recovered fully, and thankfully, she never repeated the behavior.

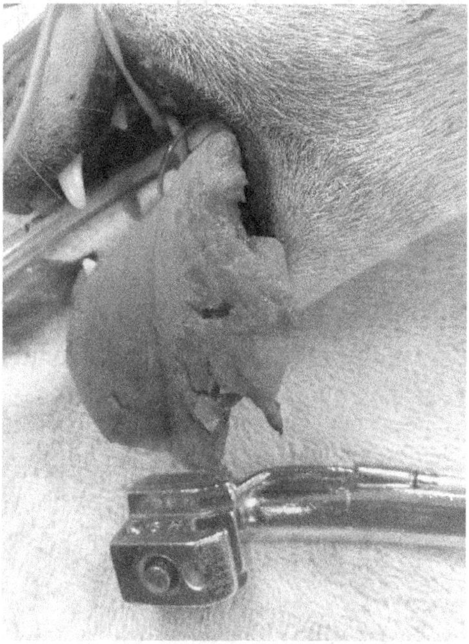

Figure 10

Finally, there's the story of a young dog who had an unfortunate encounter with a very common household appliance. Before I continue, let me say that this can be a gruesome injury when first seen, but most dogs I've treated for this type of trauma recovered well. The culprit? A paper shredder.

If you own a paper shredder, please, go unplug it right now. These machines, especially in homes with children or pets, should only ever be plugged in when actively in use. Even if your shredder has an automatic shut-off, it should remain unplugged. I have one at home, and my dogs are locked out of the room whenever I use it—it only gets plugged in when I'm shredding something. Many dogs love to play with paper. They rip it, toss it, and sometimes even open wrapped presents, which we humans often find adorable. But that playful curiosity makes shredders especially dangerous.

Most of these injuries occur when a young dog, out of curiosity, sniffs or licks a shredder. It's harmless until something—clothing, a tongue, or a lip—gets caught as the motor starts. One unfortunate pup didn't just get her tongue stuck; her lip was also pulled in, and the shredder tore off parts of both (shown in Figure 11). She was first taken to her primary care veterinarian for repair, but due to poor blood supply to the area, the closure didn't heal, and part of the wound reopened.

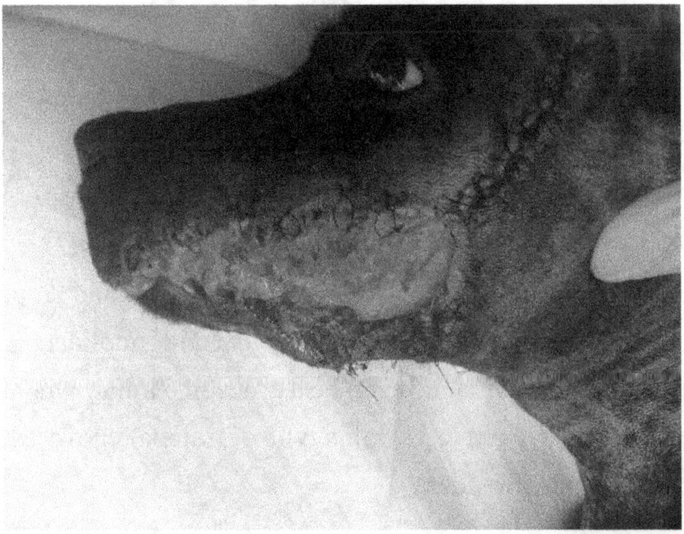

Figure 11

Because of the loss of vascular supply, we had to leave the wound open for several days, performing regular debridement to remove any dead tissue until we could attempt a delayed surgical repair. It was a complex case, and we involved one of our board-certified surgeons to help create a functional and cosmetic result. It required creativity and precision, but in the end, we achieved both. The dog made a full recovery and went on to live a happy, healthy, normal life after this terrible accident.

Chapter 5

Potpourri Of A Different Sort: Rubber Bands And Fishing Hooks!

Oh, rubber bands and fishing hooks can certainly be problems in our veterinary pets. Let's start with the first one, rubber bands. Most of the time, I would like to believe that when these are applied to pets in any way, it should be done by a professional. There is a method called banding, or elastration, that is used to castrate male goats. I don't necessarily agree with the technique, and the AVMA actually discourages its use. I won't get into all the details, but in short, it involves placing a rubber band around the base of the scrotum to cut off blood supply. Eventually, the scrotum and testicles, having lost circulation, swell at first, and then dry up and fall off. I have no doubt it's a painful procedure, and probably why it's discouraged.

But I digress, I don't really see many goats at our hospital. I do, however, occasionally see pets who have had a rubber band applied to them. Much of the time, these injuries occur when a child is playing with a pet and applies a hair tie or rubber band to their furry friend. Maybe they were playing dress-up or trying to "style" the dog's hair. Here's the kicker: if you're playing hair stylist with your dog, the dog probably has longer hair, which means a small rubber band can be easily hidden or lost within that hair. This often means the owners, or at least the parents, don't recognize that there's a problem for several days. Eventually, if the rubber band is placed around an ear or a limb, the blood supply is cut off, the skin starts to die, and an infection sets in. Owners may then either notice the pain their pet is experiencing or the smell from the infection.

I've included two such examples below. In the first, the rubber band was placed around the ear of a dog (Figure 12), and you can see that the edges of the ear are essentially gone because the tissue died off from the pressure. The tip of the ear is swollen, red, and compromised. In the picture, the dog's eye is on the bottom left, and she's wearing a muzzle. Don't worry, we had already given her pain medication. You can clearly see the line where the rubber band was placed. We actually had to amputate part of this dog's ear under anesthesia, and of course, she received pain medication and antibiotics. She recovered well in the long term, but ouch, what a thing to go through.

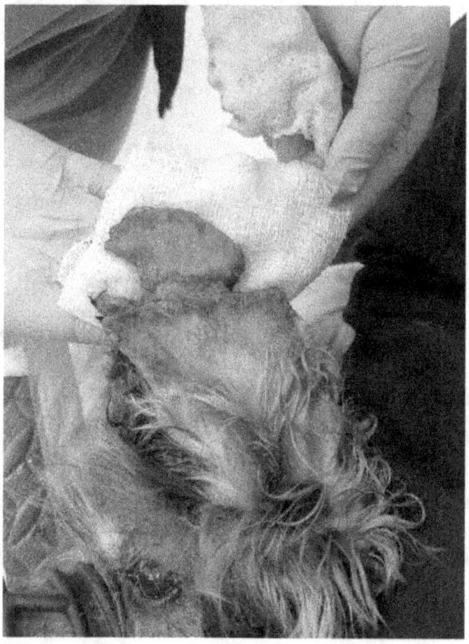

Figure 12

The second picture (Figure 13) shows the back of a dog's neck; her ears are toward the upper right of the image. She had been wearing a stretchy collar that was left on too long as she grew, resulting in a deep cut almost all the way around her neck. Sometimes, we see similar injuries from collars that were placed on young animals and never adjusted as they grew up. This dog just needed the collar removed and some basic wound care, including pain medication and antibiotics, and she healed up just fine, though it took several weeks. A word to the wise: never use rubber bands or stretchy elastic materials like hair ties on pets, as they can cause serious injury.

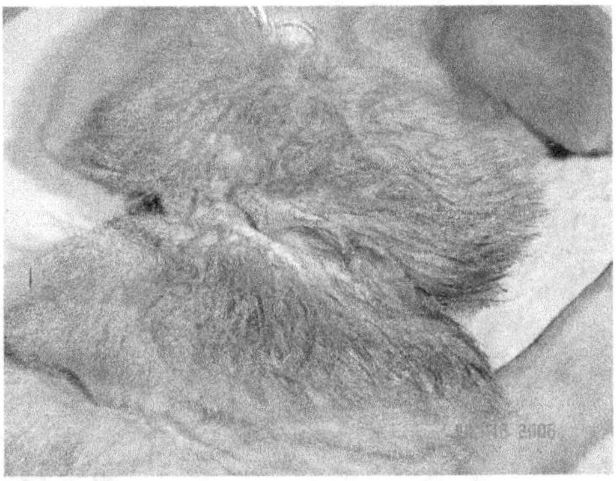

Figure 13

Ok, let's move on to something a little funnier and maybe a little less gruesome: fish hooks. It's not hard to see why both cats and dogs might be interested in fish hooks, right? Not new ones, of course, but old, used ones. They likely smell amazing to pets—covered in bits of fishy bait or guts. And if they smell good, well, they probably taste good too. To a dog or cat that loves fish, they probably seem irresistible. So, after your fishing trip with the family, don't forget to clean off those hooks and, most importantly, store them where your pets can't reach them!

The first photo shows a dog who managed to get a three-pronged fishing hook caught in its lip and tongue (Figure 14). Ouch! Owners often try to remove these at home, but there are a couple of important things to keep in mind when trying to remove something from your pet. First, they're painful, and most animals are not going to sit still while you pull a fish hook out of their mouth, nose, or tongue. They'll thrash and flail, making removal dangerous. That's why at the veterinary hospital, one of our favorite mantras applies: "Better living through chemistry!" We have all sorts of safe, fast-acting medications to ease pain and calm the animal, allowing us to quickly and safely remove the hook. Many of these medications wear off quickly or are reversible, so pets are usually ready to go home in no time.

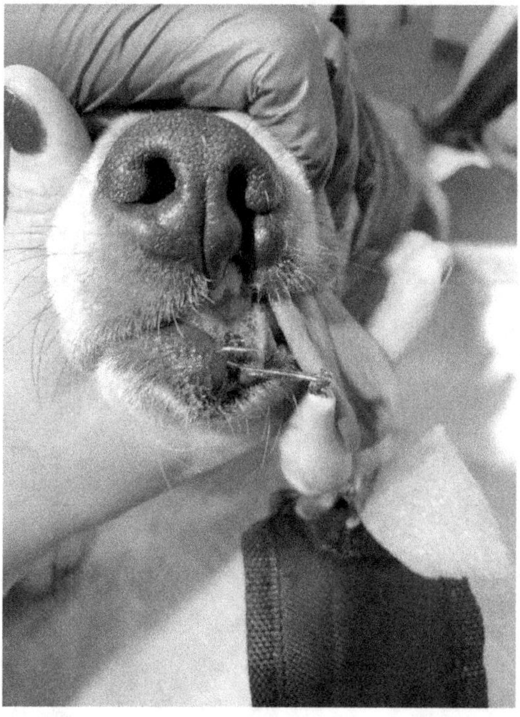

Figure 14

The second thing to know is that fish hooks usually can't come out the same way they went in. They have little reverse-facing barbs that prevent the hook from slipping out—great for catching fish, not so great for your dog's lip. So, you can't just pull on them. We usually have to push the hook all the way through the tissue until the barb comes out the other side, then cut off the tip with wire cutters before sliding the remaining portion back out safely. Easy-peezy!

Back to that first photo, the dog had a three-pronged lure, and two prongs were stuck through different parts of the lips. As a side note, you can see that this dog also had a cleft nose and lip on the right side of the picture (left side of the dog). She had been living with it for quite some time with no adverse effects.

The second picture (Figure 15) shows a cat who, for the same reason, got a small hook attached to her upper lip. The third picture (Figure 16) features a black Labrador who must have only been interested in the smell, not the taste, because she managed to get a hook stuck in her nose! Admittedly, this one was a little funny to us—she came into the treatment area jingling, and we could hear her nose from about a hundred feet away.

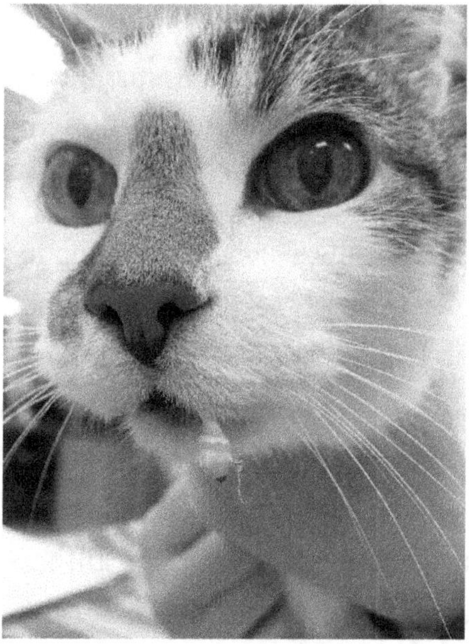

Figure 15

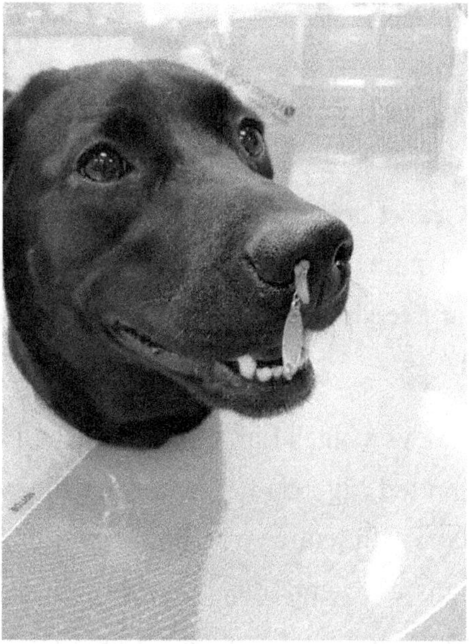

Figure 16

In all these cases, as I mentioned, it's an easy fix. A little sedation, push the hook through, clip off the end, clean the wound, and they do fine. All of these pets went home within a short time after coming to the ER.

However, there's always one more thing to consider. If you cut yourself on a rusty piece of metal, what does the doctor do? They ask about your last tetanus shot. Clostridium tetani is an anaerobic bacterium that lives on old or dirty metal and can cause a dangerous infection. The bacteria produce a neurotoxin that interferes with normal muscle movement, leading to lockjaw. Dogs and cats are more resistant to tetanus than people, but we still take precautions. Since pets don't get tetanus shots, we treat them with antibiotics to prevent the bacteria from growing and producing toxins. So, even if you manage to remove a fish hook at home, please follow up with your veterinarian to ensure your pet gets antibiotics to prevent infection.

Tetanus looks a little different in dogs and cats than in people. They tend to get muscle contracture in the face and head, causing lockjaw so they can't open their mouths. They can recover over time, but they'll need pain medication, muscle relaxers, and sometimes even a temporary feeding tube so they can eat and drink while the toxin wears off.

Figure 17 shows a black Lab mix who actually developed tetanus. Her ears were pulled high on her head, her lips were drawn back in what looked like a grin (called a sardonic grin), and her jaw wouldn't open. These signs are temporary, and though medications can help manage symptoms, the neurological effects can last several weeks.

You can see we placed a temporary feeding tube through her nose, called a nasogastric tube, so we could feed her while she recovered.

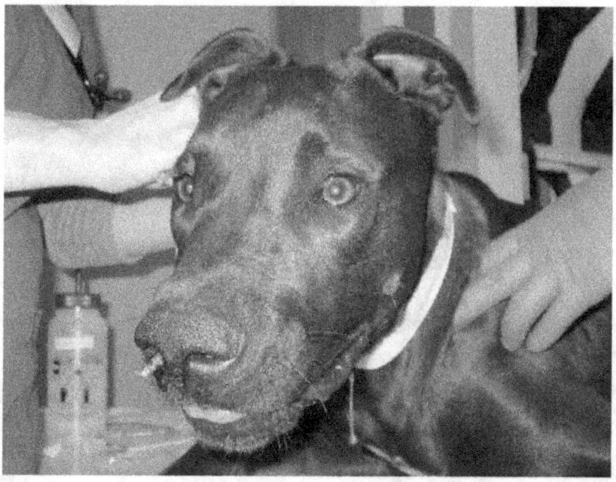

Figure 17

Many times, when tetanus occurs in pets, the original wound is so small that owners didn't even notice it. Even a tiny thorn or a small fish hook can do it. By the time the signs appear, the wound has often healed. Luckily, this doesn't happen very often.

Finally, whenever we know a pet has been exposed to fish hooks, we always ask if there might be more missing. We often take x-rays of the neck, chest, and stomach to check for other hooks inside the patient. Sometimes we have to retrieve them with an endoscope. The final picture of this chapter (Figure 18) shows a radiograph of a dog who had swallowed a fishing hook, which we removed endoscopically. You'd think it would be a simple procedure, but if there's a lot of food in the stomach, it's like finding a needle in a mud pile with tweezers—not easy! And you have to be careful to grasp the hook properly or it can snag tissue on the way out.

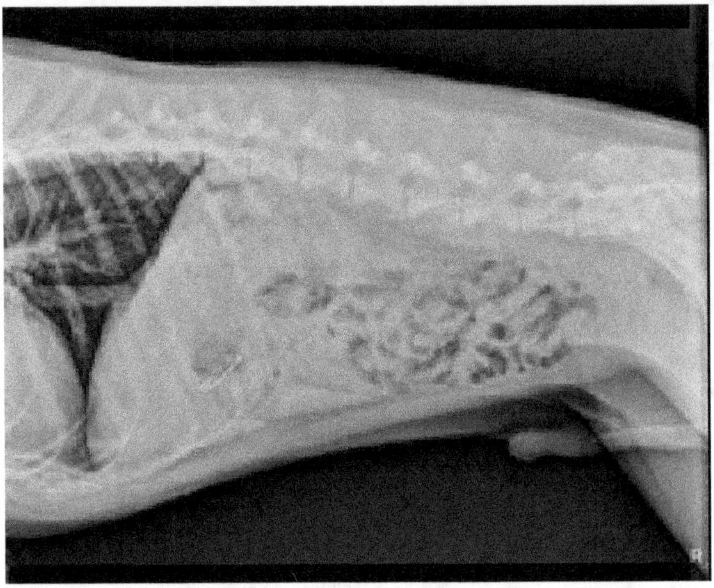

Figure 18

Chapter 6

The trouble of the tiny testicles

I have seen so many problems involving tiny testicles in this profession. Most of these issues seem to occur in juvenile animals whose testicles do not descend properly, but that is only the beginning of the troubles.

I'll start this set of stories with something that happened during my internship. It was one of the first patients I ever saw on emergency, and I was a little dumbfounded by what I was finding. If you were watching from a distance, you could probably hear the gears in my head turning as I tried to figure out what to do. The young dog I was seeing had gone to its primary care veterinarian earlier in the day for a neuter. The owners reported that both testicles had been removed, although they had not fully descended into the scrotum and were located in the inguinal region or groin, essentially the armpit of the hind limb.

That part is not unusual. Testicles start off in the abdomen and usually descend fully into the scrotum by the time a dog or cat is a few months old. The artery, vein, and spermatic cord lengthen as the testicles move out of the abdomen through a canal in the groin and into their final destination, the scrotum. Sometimes they stop in the inguinal region, and sometimes they never make it out of the abdomen, a condition we call cryptorchidism.

When performing a neuter on a dog with inguinal testicles, the surgery itself is not particularly complicated. Instead of making a single incision in front of, near, or around the scrotum as in a typical neuter procedure, the incision is made in the lateral groin region on either side of the penis over each testicle. You can usually feel the testicles under the skin, and they are often quite accessible in this region. The surgery is not much different from a regular neuter, except that there is one incision per testicle on each side of the penis in the groin, a few inches apart depending on the size of the patient.

However, in this case, I am not sure whether the veterinarian performing the surgery was unfamiliar with this type of procedure or simply inexperienced, but they decided to make a single incision instead of the two that would normally be required to remove both testicles. The incision was made directly over one testicle. Instead of creating a second incision, the veterinarian reached across from the first incision under the skin to the opposite side of the abdomen to pull the other testicle over to the same side as the incision for removal. This is not something you are supposed to do, and not something I have ever seen before or since.

The recently neutered dog presented to me on the emergency service straining to urinate but unable to pass any urine. Urinary obstruction is something we see quite commonly in veterinary medicine, often due to stones or crystals that block the urethra, the tube through which urine exits the body. The urethra begins in the urinary bladder and exits through the penis. When it is obstructed, animals strain to urinate but cannot pass any urine, which quickly becomes a medical emergency. Not only is it painful, but if the animal is completely obstructed, urine backs up into the kidneys, and toxins that are normally excreted begin to accumulate in the bloodstream.

We worry most about elevated potassium, which can alter the electrical activity of the heart. A high potassium level slows the heart and, if severe enough, can stop it entirely. So, when we receive a call about an animal straining to urinate but unable to do so, we always recommend they come in immediately.

On physical examination, I could see that the inguinal incision was healing normally, but the dog was clearly straining. No urine was passing, and on palpation, I could feel that its bladder was very large, indicating an obstruction. The next step was to pass a urinary catheter, which is inserted through the tip of the penis up the urethra and into the bladder to relieve the obstruction temporarily while we investigate the cause.

However, when I passed the catheter, it only advanced a few centimeters before stopping. I tried flushing saline through it, and to my surprise, the saline came out through the neuter incision. This was confusing because the incision was several centimeters away from the penis. The only logical explanation was that during surgery, while attempting to remove both testicles through a single incision, the veterinarian had inadvertently tied off the urethra. This meant the dog was physically unable to urinate because the urethra had been ligated.

This was a major medical error and needed immediate correction. Surgery on the urethra is complex and should only be performed by a board-certified surgeon to minimize complications, which can be serious. I knew the dog would need to see our surgeon the following day. That evening, we administered pain medication, and I temporarily alleviated the obstruction by performing a cystocentesis, inserting a needle through the skin into the bladder to drain it. We closely monitored the dog's vital signs and electrolytes, including blood potassium, overnight.

The next day, one of our veterinary surgeons performed a urethral repair. The dog recovered well and was discharged a few days later, urinating normally. It was a very stressful case for me. I was a new veterinarian but recognized an error committed by another doctor and was unsure how to proceed. I consulted with my hospital manager, and together with the surgeon, we called the other veterinarian to discuss the situation. Naturally, the veterinarian was mortified by the mistake and covered the cost of the dog's care.

The next testicle-related case I saw was somewhat similar. Another juvenile dog had been brought in for a standard neuter. When the dog arrived for surgery, only one testicle was present in the scrotum. The attending veterinarian could not feel the other testicle in either the scrotum or the inguinal region, correctly assuming it was still inside the abdomen. That is the most common location when a testicle has not descended.

The veterinarian proceeded logically, exploring the abdominal cavity, but still found no second testicle. The surgery went well, and the dog recovered uneventfully. The patient was referred to our hospital to help determine where the missing testicle might be and whether it was truly present. It is extremely rare for an animal to have only one testicle, but it is possible. I have even performed ultrasounds on three dogs (over a 20 year time frame) that had only one kidney, so such anomalies do occur.

I perform many diagnostic ultrasounds at our hospital, typically to identify pathology in animals showing symptoms like vomiting or to clarify findings on x-rays. It is rare for me to use ultrasound to locate a normal structure that may simply be in an abnormal position, such as a testicle inside the abdomen.

When this dog arrived, I was asked to examine its abdomen with ultrasound to locate the missing testicle. I was unsure how successful I would be, as I had not done this specific type of search before. Normally, testicles are easily visible within the scrotum in healthy adult dogs. They have a distinct appearance on ultrasound, but I was skeptical that I could locate one inside the abdomen, especially since the doctor had failed to find it in surgery!

I carefully examined the entire abdominal cavity with my ultrasound machine, searching for the missing testicle. I also scanned the small remaining scrotum, as it is not typically removed in juvenile neuters, but found nothing there either. I went through all possible locations, knowing that having only one testicle is exceedingly rare. Finally, I checked the inguinal region, and there it was, seated deep within the tissue.

As it turned out, only one testicle had fully descended into the scrotum, while the other was lodged deep in the inguinal region. Even after locating it with ultrasound, we could not feel it through palpation, nor could the referring veterinarian during surgery. The dog was sent back to its primary care veterinarian, who successfully removed the second testicle. It was a reminder that veterinarians are human, and even when errors occur, they can often be corrected. The dog did very well.

The final "tiny testicle" story involves a five-month-old male dog scheduled for neutering in about a month. He presented to our emergency clinic because he was in pain. This dog was old enough that both testicles had descended into the scrotum, so this was not a case of undescended testicles. However, he showed signs of significant abdominal discomfort.

Because he was young, we first suspected that he might have eaten something inappropriate, perhaps a foreign object causing abdominal pain. The owner denied any history of that, and there was no evidence of trauma, such as a fall or being kicked.

On examination, everything appeared normal except for the dog's very high heart rate, likely from pain localized to the caudal abdomen. We administered pain medication and re-examined him to help identify the source of the pain. Once the referred pain subsided, it became clear that one testicle was the source. It was about 25 percent larger than the other, firmer, and extremely painful to touch.

Although the pain medication helped, his heart rate remained high. I decided to ultrasound the testicle to determine if there was trauma or another abnormality. The ultrasound revealed an enlarged testicle with fluid surrounding it and, using color flow Doppler, I could see that blood flow was severely diminished. This was highly suspicious for testicular torsion, where the testicle twists on its own blood supply, cutting off circulation, leading to swelling, pain, and eventual tissue death. This is a very rare condition in dogs (I've only ever seen two in my career!)

This is also one of the rare instances where an emergency neuter is the recommended treatment. I contacted our on-call surgeon, since this was not a procedure I had performed before. At first, he didn't believe my diagnosis, but I convinced him of my findings, and he came in to operate. The surgical findings confirmed a testicular torsion. I took a photo of the abnormal testicle for reference, shown in Figure 19. Normally, a testicle is light pink and fleshy, but this one was swollen, congested, and bruised. I cannot imagine how much discomfort this dog was in, and I was very glad we were able to quickly diagnose and treat the problem.

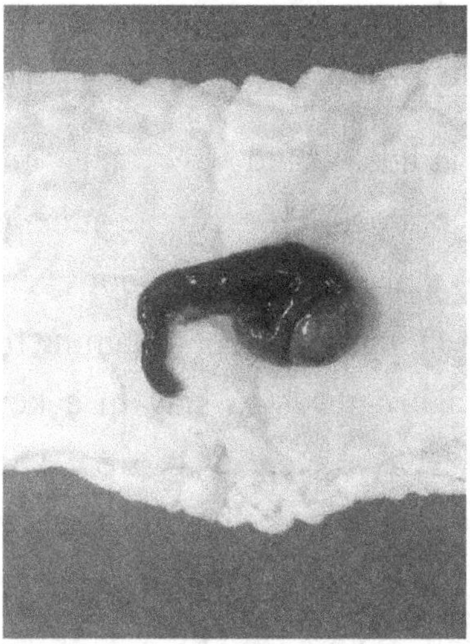

Figure 19

Chapter 7

Little help? AKA How did you manage to do that?

Dogs do manage to get themselves into some ridiculous situations. Sometimes they're serious, and sometimes they're just plain silly. One of the more common toy-related injuries we see occurs when a marrow bone gets stuck on a dog's jaw.

Most veterinarians would argue that marrow bones are not particularly good for dogs. They can be quite hard on the teeth, that's for sure. I'll admit that I've given my dogs some of these bones over the years. They're a long-lasting, entertaining treat, and can be refilled with food when a pet needs to stay in a kennel for a few hours. Recently, though, I've moved away from large marrow bones and started using dog-specific toys, like thick rubber Kong-style toys that can easily be filled with food. They're flexible, refillable, and gentle on the teeth. I highly recommend them.

A number of years ago, I had a very large Pitbull named Milton. He's part of the reason I love the Pitbull breed so much, and also why I have a soft spot for white dogs with brown spots, even when they can be a little naughty. Milton was definitely a toy chewer, and when you have a 90-pound pittie with a massive jaw who loves to destroy toys, you become very selective about which ones are worth buying.

I once purchased a Kong-brand toy, though I can't even remember which type it was. I was disappointed that it didn't hold up as well as advertised for "tough chewers." I gave it to Milton, and in less than an hour, it was completely destroyed. Frustrated with my purchase, I did what any Canadian who grew up in the 80s would do—I wrote a letter to the company to let them know how easily the toy had been chewed apart.

Being the responsible company they are, Kong quickly refunded my money. The refund came with a letter that read, "Dear Dr. Linklater, we are sorry to hear that our product did not stand up to your dog's obviously very impressive chewing habits." It went on to say, "Given your credentials, reputation, and your dog, we would like to invite you to participate in our toy testing program."

The short version of that story is that Kong offered to send me monthly installments of dog toys at no cost, asking only that I provide feedback on how well they held up and whether Milton enjoyed them. We happily agreed, and for several months, our house filled up with toys. Some lasted, some didn't, but we had fun testing and reporting on them.

One of the toys we received was a Jolly Pets Tug-n-Toss toy—but it was the version made for horses, so it was rather large. Essentially, it's a rubber ball with a built-in handle. Milton loved that toy and played with it endlessly. It started his lifelong obsession with balls, which, as it turned out, led to more than one trip to the veterinary hospital. That story, though, might be best saved for another time. Milton was one of the reasons I became comfortable treating my own pets, something not all veterinarians are entirely at ease with. He helped build my confidence as a specialist in more ways than one.

But I digress. Back to marrow bones. I don't have a problem with owners giving their dogs marrow bones, though I personally don't treat dental issues, so it's best to check with your primary care veterinarian for their opinion. My only recommendation is to make sure the bones are long—at least four inches. The longer the better. If they're too short, less than three inches or so, there's a real risk that they can get stuck on the lower jaw, as shown below in Figure 20.

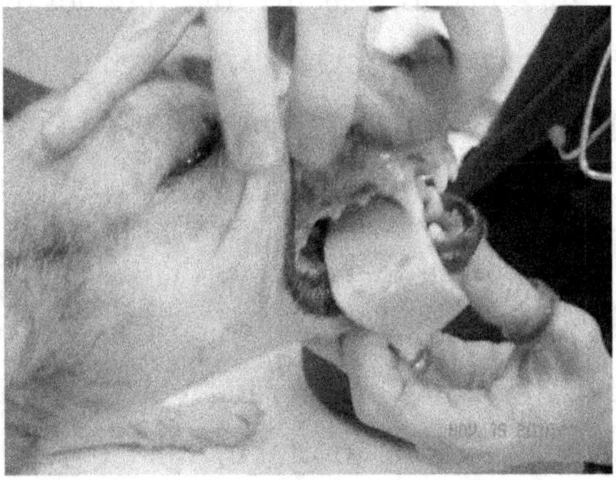

Figure 20

There are several ways to remove a stuck bone. Sometimes we can simply twist it back over the tip of the jaw and it pops right off. Other times, owners bring their dogs in after they've been in a kennel all day, unsupervised, with the bone stuck for hours. By then, the swelling can make removal much more difficult. In those cases, we often need to sedate the dog and remove the bone using large lock-cutters, a hacksaw, a bone saw, or a cast-cutting (oscillating) saw, which can sometimes cause further injury. So, let that be a gentle word of caution—best to prevent these situations when possible.

Sometimes, when dogs are left alone in their kennels—especially those with separation anxiety—they can get themselves into trouble with the kennel itself. My own dog, Ella, whom I've mentioned before, had terrible separation anxiety. She chewed and broke out of several metal wire kennels, often causing minor injuries to herself. I was fortunate to have family support for most of her life, so she rarely needed to be left in a kennel. I'm grateful every day that my current dogs actually love their kennels.

Not all dogs are so lucky. A couple of dogs pictured below weren't particularly happy with their kennel situations and managed to get themselves stuck. The silver lining, at least, was that because their faces were wedged into the kennel bars, they couldn't bite us during their rescue. The downside was that it was probably quite painful for them, and they likely never liked their kennels again—not that they were big fans to begin with!

The first was a middle-aged dachshund known to be a cage biter. The owner kenneled him for the day and left for work. When they returned, the poor pooch had locked his jaw and teeth around the kennel's locking mechanism and couldn't get free (Figure 21). His jaw had become swollen, and the tissue was starting to envelop the metal bars. Even after removing the door from the rest of the kennel, we couldn't get the door off the dog, so we had to sedate him and cut it free.

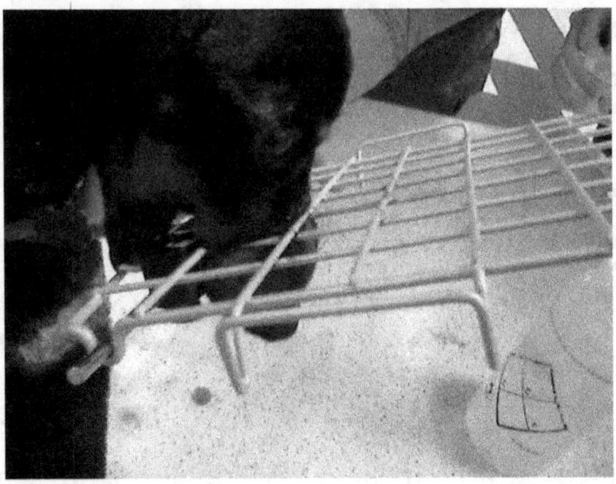

Figure 21

A similar story unfolded with our next patient, a young, cage-biting Shih Tzu mix who came in stuck to her kennel. She had the common black wire kennel that often comes with a small divider panel used to adjust the size as a puppy grows. These dividers have little hooks on one end, and she managed to pull one of them into the kennel and started chewing on it. The hook got caught in her mouth, and before long, her face was stuck to the kennel (Figure 22). Her poor little face was all smooshed up, and she was clearly uncomfortable. She needed pain medication before we could remove the divider safely.

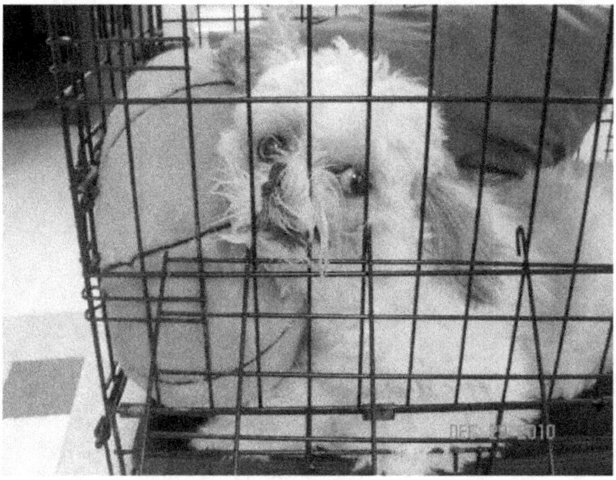

Figure 22

Thankfully, all these dogs did well. They went home on pain medications for a few days, and in some cases, antibiotics if there were any breaks in the skin. Still, let's be cautious and try to avoid these kinds of injuries in the first place.

And so ends the first round of *Tails from the ICU!*

I hope you enjoyed this book and some of the trials and tribulations of an emergency room veterinarian. I'm currently writing the next installment of *Tails from the ICU*. Be safe, love your pets, and be kind to one another.

Andrew Linklater, DVM, DACVECC

www.ingramcontent.com/pod-product-compliance
Lightning Source LLC
LaVergne TN
LVHW052243200926
848481LV00002B/258
* 9 7 9 8 2 3 3 9 5 3 9 1 0 *